When
Antibiotics
Fail

When Antibiotics Fail

Restoring the Ecology of the Body

Marc Lappé

North Atlantic Books
Berkeley, California

When Antibiotics Fail: Restoring the Ecology of the Body

Copyright © 1986, 1988, 1995 by North Atlantic Books. No portion of this book, except for brief review, may be reproduced in any form without written permission of the publisher. For information contact North Atlantic Books.

North Atlantic Books
P.O. Box 12327
Berkeley, CA 94712

Cover photo of malaria-infected blood sample by James Galvin
Cover design by Paula Morrison
Printed in the United States of America by Malloy Lithographing

When Antibiotics Fail: Restoring the Ecology of the Body is sponsored by the Society for the Study of Native Arts and Sciences, a nonprofit educational corporation whose goals are to develop an educational and crosscultural perspective linking various scientific, social, and artistic fields; to nurture a holistic view of the arts, sciences, humanities, and healing; and to publish and distribute literature on the relationship of mind, body, and nature.

Library of Congress Cataloging-in-Publication Data

Lappé, Marc
      When antibiotics fail : restoring the ecology of the body / Marc
Lappé.
           p.   cm.
      Originally published in 1986.
      Includes bibliographical references and index.
      ISBN 1-55643-191-0 (pbk.)
      1. Antibiotics.   2. Drug resistance in microorganisms.
3. Antibiotics—Effectiveness.   I. Title.
RM267.L37 1995
615'329—dc20   94-48258
                                                                          CIP

For my mother

Acknowledgments

Perhaps unlike most books on technical subjects, this list of acknowledgments is short, but nonetheless heartfelt. My very special thanks to Loretta Barrett, Executive Editor of Doubleday/ Anchor Press, for suggesting the idea of a book on antibiotics. Early research was done by Roger Smith, M.S. Typing of rough manuscripts was ably and generously done by Leslie Henriques. Final editing and review were done by Nichol Lovera, my wife, who supported my efforts with love and understanding over the period of conceiving and writing this book. Debra Jan Bibel, Ph.D., a microbiologist in her own right, provided many of the illustrations and gave generously of her time in editing the book for technical accuracy. Of course, final responsibility for the overall content of the book rests with me alone.

Contents

Foreword

In the early 1980s, a silent menace was emerging, which individual doctors had observed, but the field of medicine as a whole was slow to recognize. The general public seemed wholly unaware. I had been seeing patients whose health I believed had been compromised by the phenomenon. As I searched the medical literature, I found few resources that addressed a new problem in medicine: common bacteria which should have been defeated by antibiotics seemed strangely resistant.

The search led me to *When Antibiotics Fail,* published by Dr. Marc Lappé in 1986. This illuminating and pioneering work described problems resulting from antibiotic overuse which disrupted the natural ecologies of the body. *When Antibiotics Fail* warned that antibiotics could kill off micro-organisms necessary to fight infection in the healthy body, lowering the immune system's resistance.

Dr. Lappé painted a startling picture of our dependence on "miracle drugs" like penicillin, and of the immunologic consequences of overprescribing antibiotics. A biologist active in toxicology, hazard evaluation systems, and health policy, Dr. Lappé carefully described how antibiotics and resistance work, and what constitutes inappropriate use of antibiotics. His message highlighted the arrogance with which we often regard nature and our own abilities to control it. Since Dr. Lappé's book was first published, the antibiotic crisis has continued to grow.

In 1977, the Surgeon General of the United States stated that it was "time to close the book on infectious diseases." Many physicians believed that it was only a matter of time before infections would be a thing of the past. Unfortunately, the microbial world has rebounded with vigor. In 1992, the Institute of Medicine authored a report entitled *Emerging Infections: Microbial Threats to Health in the United States* which stated that "Pathogenic microbes can be resilient, dangerous foes. Although it is impossible to predict their individual emergence in time and place, we can be confident that new microbial diseases will emerge."

What has caused this dramatic shift in outlook? The shift has occurred because doctors have witnessed a startling increase in diseases once easily treated with antibiotics. Drugs such as penicillin have become impotent in the face of more virulent strains of common bacteria. One strain of bacteria, it is supposed, may be passing its tools for antibiotic resistance to other species of bacteria. Physicians have stood by helplessly as hospitalized patients died for lack of an effective antimicrobial. They have watched the emergence of immunosuppressive diseases such as AIDS change the ground rules for dealing with infectious organisms. All told, modern physicians may be witness to the most dramatic shift in infectious disease since the introduction of penicillin decades ago. The major difference is that in 1941 penicillin heralded a new age of success against infectious disease. Today, we face an ominous threat brought about by many of the same microbes once thought under control.

The issue of antibiotic resistance has gained widespread attention. The senior scientific advisor at the National Institutes of Health has declared that "we have an epidemic of microbial resistance." Harold C. Neu, physician and professor of pharmacology at Columbia University, wrote in *Science*, August, 1992, that in 1941 we could cure a patient with pneumococcal pneumonia by giving them 40,000 units of penicillin per day for four days. Today, we could give a patient 24 million units of penicillin and he or she still might die of pneumococcal meningitis. Officials at the Centers for Disease Control and Prevention have stated that "the post-antimicrobial era may be rapidly approaching in which untreatable infections will again be seen."

For example, in January 1994, the CDC reported on an epidemic of resistant pneumococcal infections in rural Memphis and Kentucky. The bugs had spread through day care centers "like a chain letter," leaving toddlers with ear infections, pneumonia, and six cases of meningitis.

Reports in both the medical and popular literature have noted world-

wide concern raised by the specter of infectious disease and the growing impotence of once-effective drugs to combat them:

- *Time,* August 28, 1992: "Attack of The Superbugs"

- *Newsweek,* March 28, 1994: "Cover Story: The End of
  Antibiotics"

- *Time,* August 19, 1994: "Revenge of the Killer Microbes: Are
  We Losing the Battle Against Infectious Disease?"

- Annals of Internal Medicine, September 1993: "The Conquest
  of Infectious Disease: Who Are We Kidding?"

Dr. Lappé's descriptions of the consequences of hormones and
antibiotics used in the feedlot and in fertilizer have been corroborated
by later research in the early 1990s. An analysis done by the U.S.
Congress' General Accounting Office identified traces of sixty-four
different antibiotics in cow's milk at levels "that raise health concerns." Antibiotic levels deemed safe by the Food and Drug Administration have been shown by scientists at Rutgers University to
increase the rate at which resistant bacteria emerged by 600 to 2,700
percent.

Antibiotics used in animal husbandry have apparently caused the
emergence of antibiotic-resistant microbes in family farmers, which
can then be passed on to the community. In a study conducted by
Tufts University, tetracycline given to chicks caused development of
antibiotic-resistant strains of *E. coli.* after only a few days. During
the next three months, the bacteria developed resistance to multiple
antibiotics including ampicillin and streptomycin, even though these
drugs had not been given. Over the next six months, the farmers har-
bored *E. coli* with the same resistance pattern. In a related study conducted in Germany, antibiotic resistance was passed from pigs, to
farmers, and disturbingly, to members of the community who merely
lived in the area.

Stuart Levy, M.D., of Tufts University School of Medicine has
pointed out in *The Antibiotic Paradox* that manure of antibiotic-treated
animals as fertilizer introduces antibiotic-resistant bacteria into the
soil. These microbes may survive and be carried on fertilized fruits
and vegetables, affecting even those who eat no animal products.

Dr. Lappé has highlighted the problem of hospital-acquired infection and the serious threat these infections pose to life. The issue has if anything become more urgent. In 1989, only one New York hospital reported vancomycin-resistant enterococcus. In 1991, thirty-eight hospitals reported vancomycin-resistant strains. This is alarming, since vancomycin represents the last stand against this organism.

In 1994, Dr. Ronald Jones and others from the University of Iowa collected samples from forty-three hospitals across the United States. They found that about 16 percent of the enterococci can withstand vancomycin and roughly half of these are also resistant to all the other primary antibiotics used against them. These antibiotic-resistant microbes are even resistant to some drugs that have not yet been released for routine treatment. Antibiotic-resistant enterococci can cause life-threatening infection of the heart and blood. They may also pass their genes for resistance to microbes such as staph.

Jeffrey Fisher, M.D., author of *The Plague Makers*, has proposed that prolonged overuse of antibiotics to fight minor infections and act as prophylaxis in the prevention of disease, might be contributing to the development of AIDS. He bases this hypothesis on interviews with some of the top virologists in the world. Antibiotic use is high among the populations at risk to developing AIDS, as it is in the general population. Over 60 percent of intravenous drug users use prophylactic antibiotics in hopes of preventing cellulitis, phlebitis, and abscess formation. More than 40 percent of homosexual men were found to be regularly treating themselves with prescription antibiotics. According to immunologist Robert Root-Bernstein, "The irony of the situation is that in protecting themselves against everyday infections, they open themselves up to exotic and deadly infections."

Many antibiotics, in addition to fostering antibiotic resistance, are strongly immunosuppressive. This is especially true of the broad-spectrum cephalosporins such as cephalexin. It may be this combination of factors that accelerates the progression of AIDS in those with an extensive history of antibiotic use. Dr. Luc Montagnier, discoverer of the HIV virus and director of virology at the Pasteur Institute in Paris, has recently presented his findings that antibiotic overuse may cause a form of mycoplasma to revert to a more virulent form that evades treatment. This may represent one important co-factor in development of AIDS and offer a warning to those who depend too much on these powerful drugs.

In the past, medicine has had the luxury of switching to new, more powerful antibiotics when the old ones failed. Today, we do not have this luxury. Since 1990, the FDA has approved just ten new antibiotics.

Where does this leave us? It seems clear that we must chart a new course with regard to the manner in which we care for microbial disease. Thomas McKeown, noted physician and professor of social medicine and hygiene at the University of Birmingham, summed it up this way "... the conclusion which seems inescapable is that the influences which determine man's response to infectious disease—genetics, nutrition, environment, behavior, as well as medicine—are infinitely complex. We need to be very cautious before assuming that we fully understand the infection, or that we have in our hands the certain means of their control."

The Institute of Medicine's report *Emerging Infections,* published in 1992, stated that our effort to deal with emerging infections and the resistance crisis should include "adopting health-enhancing behaviors." Beyond this, they gave no indication of what these behaviors might include. We have argued in *Beyond Antibiotics* (North Atlantic Books, 1994) that at least five critical areas deserve our attention in an effort to optimize host immune defense systems. Included are diet, nutrition, lifestyle, environmental factors, and psychosocial factors. We have reviewed over 700 scientific papers that lend support to this view. By modifying personal behavior, one can improve immune function and reduce reliance upon antibiotic drugs. In addition, specific biological response modifiers can be used as immune modulators.

The issue of emerging infections and the antibiotic resistance crisis goes far beyond simple measures that regard therapeutic modifications in drug use. With the considerable amount of data available on factors that influence host immune defense and repair mechanisms, it seems only logical that this be placed at the forefront of our efforts to deal with the current crisis. We must also view this as a larger ecological issue. Can we continue to approach environmental problems and problems of human disease with a "magic bullet" mentality, or is it more prudent to address the functional needs of the human planetary organism?

It is this last view that Marc Lappé champions. It is a position that needs little justification for those of us in the field of holistic medicine, but one that needs much support to convince the orthodoxy. Dr. Lappé's case is among the most compelling to date.

Michael A. Schmidt
author of *Beyond Antibiotics*
Anoka, MN 1995

Preface

The failure of antibiotics epitomizes the paradox of too much success too soon. At the beginning of the Antibiotic Era the unique effectiveness of these drugs all but ensured that they would be overused. And this profligate use led to their undoing.

Because antibiotics were exquisitely effective for treating a few life-threatening infectious diseases like pneumonia, their application was generalized to treatable and untreatable diseases alike. Before anyone realized it, we had squandered a medical miracle. This book describes how the misuse of antibiotics occurred and the consequences of our shortsightedness. In the end, *When Antibiotics Fail* spells out what should be done to correct our failings.

LOOKING BACK

Within the decade after Alexander Fleming discovered penicillin in 1928, antibiotics were viewed as chemical wonders capable of eradicating millions of bacteria overnight. When penicillin came into widespread clinical use in the late 1940s, it was grasped by a war-weary world as a panacea for the infectious diseases that had killed more soldiers and civilians in the two World Wars than had bullets and bombs.

By the 1950s numerous antibiotics like penicillin and streptomycin were touted as the cures for virtually any kind of bacterial problem. Whole acres of farmland were sprayed with them to wrest control of crops from real or imagined microbial pests. Every conceivable pharmaceutical product from throat lozenges to baby powder was at one time or another laced with antimicrobials, often without any therapeutic rationale.

Indeed, when they worked, antibiotics were potent killers. Early formulations of penicillin could wipe out virtually any of the major infection-causing bacteria in a typical microbiology laboratory or hospital ward. Unfortunately, the most infectious organisms have changed their genetic makeup and kept pace with antibiotic inventiveness—with a vengeance.

In the beginning antibiotics did provide a therapeutic alternative to extant models of microbial prophylaxis. Certainly, they outperformed Lister's crude and noxious antiseptics and germicides in treating disease. They did so for one simple, but powerful reason: unlike the chemical disinfectants of Lister's era (circa 1867–1880), antibiotics have very little toxicity. Antiseptics like mercuric chloride, iodoform or silver nitrate readily killed bacteria on surfaces or open wounds, but they could not be injected or absorbed by the body without severe side effects.

Ironically, Alexander Fleming himself cautioned against the rush to use his miracle drug for every imaginable ill. Fleming recognized that penicillin did not kill all bacteria—and that those that survived would likely resist subsequent doses. If enough penicillin-sensitive bacteria were destroyed, Fleming realized, their successors might begin to replace the normal disease-causing bacteria as a more robust breed. His well-reasoned admonitions surely fell on deaf ears. If fact, this is the weakness of our century—an uncritical acceptance of technological breakthroughs as bounties free from harmful side-effects.

Fleming and the early microbe hunters missed another, even more critical effect: when antibiotics kill or inhibit harmful bacteria they also eliminate vast numbers of relatively benign or even beneficial bacteria. When these more benevolent counterparts die off, they leave behind a literal wasteland of vacant tissue and organs. These sites, previously occupied with normal bacteria are now free to be colonized with new ones. Some of these new ones have caused serious and previously unrecognized diseases.

The sheer magnitude of this assault is staggering. For four decades now, we have thrown hundreds of tons of antibiotics against our Hollywood imagination of microscopic enemies. In the process, we have sown seeds for a whole new array of actual germs and diseases.

UNDOING A MEDICAL MIRACLE

Our profligate use of chemotherapeutic agents has left some of us weaker than our so-called enemies. Many mammals are now plagued by a whole new order of viral and bacterial infections that were rare before the antibiotic era. Other controllable infections have become so resistant to antibiotics that only therapeutic heroics can rescue their victims. And by virtue of their antibiotic resistance, seemingly "benign" organisms that we all carry have become nightmare germs that afflict the aged, infirm, and immune-depressed.

Initially out of ignorance and now out of neglect, we have let our profligate use of antibiotics reshape the evolution of the microbial world and wrest any hope of safe management from us. Modern pharmaceuticals cannot begin to keep pace with ever newer varieties of microorganisms which emerge, like Athena from the shoulder of Zeus, fully armed to resist the latest generation of antibiotics.

But we can hardly be surprised; this has been our legacy from the almost pathetic warning of Fleming himself—that the emergence of antibiotic-resistant bacteria was inevitable. Nor can we feign surprise at the speed and breadth of the invasion of these organisms. The mutative ability of bacteria to assemble vast repertoires of resistant genes and to shuffle this knowledge indiscriminately onto wholly different microorganisms was observed dramatically at least twenty-five years ago, by Japanese researchers. As they documented the invasion of their native land by wave after wave of antibiotic-resistant diarrhea-causing bacteria, they warned an inattentive world of the folly of blind optimism in antibacterial "magic bullets."

As one antibiotic after another fell prey to bacterial resistance, the pharmaceutical giants kept one step ahead of the boom-and-bust cycle by introducing new miracle drugs at a rate of 5–10 per year. Whether by intention or omission, possibly more permanent solutions to the risk of bacterial infection such as vaccines or adjuvants that stimulate natural immune defenses were kept in the wings. An absurd pharmaceutical morality play unfolded: we became soldiers against implacable microscopic enemies with whom we actually co-evolved. Only recently have a few scientists posited that the survival of bacteria as a group underlies our own.

The medical establishment has been derelict in discerning the side effects of antibiotics. In their chemical assault on germs, antibiotics disrupt the ancient ecological balance of our own natural flora. Antibiotics can devastate the very microorganisms that maintain the homeostasis of our living internal and external surfaces. Some, like chloramphenicol, can obliterate the production of red blood cells by the bone marrow.

The same mentality that encouraged the destruction of entire Vietnamese hamlets to "save them" seemed to be at work in the early days of the antibiotic era. Massive doses of antibiotics were often used to destroy virtually all of the body's microscopic residents in order to save it from a few miscreants.

Once "cleared" of harmful and helpful bacteria alike, parts of our bodies became the aforementioned wastelands where only the most opportunistic organisms could gain a foothold and proliferate. Sometimes now, as with vaginal "yeast" infections, this overgrowth begins as a simple irritation. But in many people, the proliferation of yeast cells called *Candida albicans* ("candida" for short) runs amok, spreading system-wide disease.

Some specialists in the new medical discipline of clinical ecology believe that candida may be responsible for a range of diseases including asthma, depression, diarrhea, and even autism. While the jury is still out on these last attributions, there is no doubt that antibiotics encourage the overgrowth of candida and other undesirable pathogens.

Large numbers of unhealthful, or even disastrous organisms such as *Clostridium* (the source of the dread botulinum toxin), suddenly appear in the wake of treatments with certain antibiotics. In the intestinal tract, resistant *Clostridium* strains can release sometimes fatal toxins that annihilate the normal cellular lining of the intestinal wall and poison the patient.

ECOSYSTEM DISRUPTION

As a result of the vast present scale of antibiotic use, individuals, hospital wards as well as entire ecosystems and microenvironments have become contaminated with bacteria that resist control by antibiotics.

Antibiotics have profound effects on the populations of bacteria that live naturally on the human body. Even the most common and benign skin bacteria become resistant to further treatment following a course of antibiotics. Under special circumstances some of these bacteria can become virulent pathogens, especially in patients whose immune systems are depressed. Following simple procedures like taking blood or putting a catheter into a vein, procedures that nonetheless permit skin bacteria to enter the body, antibiotic-resistant forms like the Corynebacteria can cause intractable and sometimes fatal systemic disease.

But even a modest course of antibiotics can disrupt surface body flora sufficiently to change body odors, vaginal secretions, and the ecology of skin. Diarrhea occurs in as many as one in every 8–10 patients after some antibiotics, a reflection of the damage done internally to the normal intestinal bacteria.

These microscopic upheavals created every time we take an antibiotic have still not been fully charted. In addition to the successions of totally new populations of antibiotic-resistant cousins that spring up among bacteria, new and more robust strains of our own native bacteria also emerge from the ostensibly medicinal attacks. These mutated forms are naturally selected in perfect Darwinian fashion.

On a macroenvironmental scale, we find that acre-sized feedlots where cattle or other livestock have been laced with antibiotics are now seedbeds of human contagion, teeming with resistant bacteria. Sewage ponds, rivers, or estuaries draining feedlots have similarly become unexpected repositories of bacteria that resist the most common antibiotics. Fish and wildfowl that inhabit such contaminated waterways readily pick up and transfer the resistant bacteria to human hosts. More ominously, new data suggest that these bacteria can transmit the information for resistance to other microorganisms.

The existence of a genetic memory for antibiotic resistance in the omnipresent bacteria of these feed lots (or, for that matter, our own intestinal tracts) ominously ensures the failure of our present approach. We are breeding far more "germs" than medicines, as each new antibiotic brings into being literally millions of microscopic Benedict Arnolds. Long after the antibiotics themselves are gone from our body, these surviving bacterial traitors stand ready to spread the genetic news to all disease-causing bacteria—"This is how to mount effective resistance against the new weapons." Whole varieties, so armed by nature, seem suddenly to appear.

The resultant organisms are no playthings. Many of them bear the same disease-causing properties as the germs that they have replaced. Others pose a long-term risk no one has fully assessed, but that almost certainly threatens some of the present generation of presumably "antibiotic-safe" Americans.

Resistance to antibiotics has spread to so many different, and such unanticipated types of bacteria, that the only fair appraisal is that we have succeeded in upsetting the balance of nature. The microbes of greatest concern to man are now more diverse, more virulent, and more resistant to our therapeutic controls than ever before. Literally dozens of different infectious organisms have slipped the fetters of antibiotic control. Still other previously benign bacteria have developed greater disease-changing proclivities and wider host ranges since we challenged them with antibiotics.

CASUAL USE

These disastrous and unintended consequences of antibiotic use should have red-flagged casual treatment. Instead, antibiotics continue to be overused and overprescribed. In some countries like Mexico and Brazil, potent antibiotics have been freely available for purchase "over the counter" without a prescription.

In the United States physicians remain among the worst offenders. Some prescribe bacteria-specific antibiotics for colds or sore throats that are almost certainly virally caused, while others use antibiotics as a dubious "cover" for clean surgical procedures.

While this last use has its place (such as in heart valve surgery or certain orthopedic procedures), overuse of so-called prophyllactic antibiotics is one of the reasons hospitals are particularly plagued by antibiotic-resistant infections.

Given this professional oversight, it is little wonder that patients take antibiotics so lightly. Casual use is even more dangerous than medically indicated courses of treatment, for incomplete treatment is more apt to leave behind resistant bacteria. But given the ability of bacteria to exchange resistance information, even a life-saving prescription for one patient can create a life-threatening situation for the next.

RECOGNIZING A DILEMMA

The fact that the same treatment that saves an individual patient can jeopardize future patients epitomizes the ethical dilemma of patient-oriented medicine. In the case of antibiotic-resistant microorganisms, exclusive attention to each individual may be at the accumulating expense of the community. The consequences of this narrow view are apparent in the emergence and spread of particular diseases.

Gonorrhea is a case in point. The pattern of emergence of first penicillin-resistant and later penicillin-destroying *Neisseria gonorrhoeae* bacteria is a direct result of both chronic overprescription and poor case management.

In the last 6–7 years, this new, penicillin-destroying variant of gonorrhea has swept the globe. From just two tiny epicenters of infection, strains of a penicillinase-producing form of *Neisseria gonorrhoeae* (PPNG for short) have spread to all fifty states and Canada. Statistics from the U.S. Center for Disease Control show that PPNG gonorrhea have doubled from 1983 to 1984 to almost 7,000 cases. Canada, previously free of this dangerous pathogen, reported a 335 percent increase in the same period.

Still further evolution of antibiotic resistance has occurred since 1976 when PPNG were first recognized in the U.S. By 1983, researchers had detected gonorrhea organisms with a chromosomally carried set of data that gave *Neisseria gonorrhoeae* unprecedented resistance to penicillin, tetracycline, and the two most commonly used alternative antibiotics, erythromycin and trimethoprim-sulfa-methoxazole. The CDC and clinicians are currently collectively holding their breath that gonorrhea will remain susceptible to spec-tinomycin, virtually the last remaining alternative.

These statistics underscore a little recognized fact: we are facing a frightening series of epidemics of sexually transmitted diseases that owe their ascendancy in whole or part to the effects of chronic and ineffective use of antibiotics. In addition to gonorrhea, sex-ually transmitted diseases like *Chlamydia trichomatis,* candida, and gential herpes have all increased in exponential fashion in recent years.

Among these, the acquired immune deficiency sydrome (AIDS) is the most visible. While AIDS itself is caused by a virus, preexist-ing bacterial or parasitic diseases like malaria greatly increase the expression of the disease. Once underway, the destruction of the immune system by the AIDS virus leaves the body vulnerable to the explosive outgrowth of opportunistic infections. These infec-tions owe most of their lethality to their intractability to treatment with common antibiotics.

The organisms that thrive in AIDS patients are a bizarre and mixed lot that capitalize on the absence of normal host defenses. The most common infections are antibiotic-resistant bacteria that cause disseminated food poisoning *(Salmonella typhimurium),* pneumonia *(Pneumocystis carinii),* tuberculosis, and toxoplasmo-sis. In AIDS patients our inability to rein in these often florid in-fections with antibiotics alone points up a key deficiency in our models of disease: we fail to acknowledge that it is the *body* which ultimately controls infection, not chemicals. Without underlying immunity, drugs are meaningless.

Antibiotics can aggravate this dilemma by destroying many bac-teria that normally afford protection against some that cause serious skin and intestinal infections (streptococcus and salmonella). At the same time, these very bacteria have become more prevalent and resistant to treatment.

The emergence of antibiotic-resistant staph infections is another dramatic example of ineffective antibiotic use at the patient level.

In the 1950s, thousands of hospitals became colonized with *Staphylococcus aureus* organisms resistant to pencillin. Continuing misuse spawned multiply resistant staph that could withstand almost all of the major antibiotics. By the 1970s, outbreaks of antibiotic-resistant staph swept entire wards in hospitals in Europe, the United States, Ireland, Australia and Greece.

Many of these infections proved fatal, unstoppable by even newer antibiotics like vancomycin. Misuse escalated with the introduction of methicillin, a penicillin-like antibiotic that was immune to the penicillin-destroying enzyme made by the staphylococci. Almost universal use of this new penicillin ensured that antibiotic control of staph infections would be a brief episode in the history of our species. Optimism that we had won the battle over staph by using methicillin thus proved short-lived. After a quiescent period in the mid-1970s, when epidemic staph infections seemed to die back, these organisms staged a resurgence in the 1980s.

It is not as if clinical researchers had ignorantly neglected the underlying problem of antibiotic resistance. For methicillin-resistant infections alone, over 250 articles were published between 1960 and 1982. But the medical establishment systematically underestimated the ability of this organism to survive chemotherapeutic attacks. Hospitals failed to monitor adequately the ability of surviving organisms to "overwinter" in protected environments, and epidemiologists downplayed the role of chronic carriers of antibiotic-resistant strains of staph in transmitting disease.

While many hospitals devised effective strategies to isolate patients from these carriers, no regulatory agency insisted on routine management to limit the ultimately global spread of infection. Instead, they mandated infectious-disease surveillance committees which had little or no police power within the hospital bureaucracy. A chronic pattern of overprescription and poor patient compliance has virtually guaranteed the continual re-emergence of antibiotic-resistant organisms in any hospital environment where antibacterials are routinely prescribed.

NEW APPROACHES

Today, some courageous clinicians have suggested reversing this process by intentionally "seeding" parts of the body with non-disease-producing and antibiotic-sensitive bacteria. Benign strains of streptococcus are being used to displace tooth-decay-producing streptococcal organisms (*Streptococcus mutans*). The replacement microbes manufacture less acid than their counterparts, slowing tooth erosion.

Other researchers have tried using benign organisms for repopulating the skin or intestinal tract. Among the notable successes has been the intentional seeding of the skin of newborns with "safe" bacterial strains to minimize *Staphylococcus aureus* infections in nurseries.

By now, we should have taken into full account the importance of host resistance to disease-causing bacteria and the folly of relying on chemicals alone to control disease. But we have neglected time-honored and innovative ways to stimulate the body's defenses in favor of drugs that inevitably dampen it. In using antibiotics we predictably disrupt the resident microorganisms and create environments that demand still more medical attention. In sum, we remain profoundly ignorant about how to shape and adapt our strategies for controlling infections and how to minimize the downward sprial of diminishing antibiotic effectiveness.

We cannot develop public policies for protecting the public from overuse of antibiotics while still allowing physicians and livestock growers the continued freedom to use these vital drugs at will.

New strategies, both political and medical, are now critical, policies that reestablish the wisdom of the body and protect the public as a whole, and future generations of mammals, from the long-term consequences of a hit-and-run solution to a complex and many-levelled problem.

Preface to the 1988 Edition

A TARNISHED MIRACLE

When I first wrote the original version of this book under the title, *Germs That Won't Die,* I prophesied that our failure to respect the adaptability of the microbal world would lead to the global spread of antibiotic resistant bacteria. In the ten years since that was written, this prophesy has been amply fulfilled. New germs in groups that were never expected to develop antibiotic resistance have emerged. The veterinary practices of providing antibiotics intended for human use to animals has led to *proven* human outbreaks of disease. And more bacteria are resistant to antibiotics today than ever before.

All this happened under the less than watchful eye of public health bureaucrats concerned about rocking the boat with new policies (e.g., on farm antibiotic use). Well-intentioned physicians and pharmacists preoccupied with practicing defensive medicine and finding "quick fixes" to often complex and dangerous diseases have unwittingly aided these developments.

The consequences of irrational use of antibiotics are what this book is about. In spite of dramatic advances in charting new patterns of bacterial strains with antibiotic resistance, few public health officials have yet appreciated the roots of these disturbing consequences in the misuse of antibiotics themselves. The contribution of poor antibiotic practice to untreatable infections in the elderly and very young, bacterial sepsis in burn victims, and intractable opportunistic infections in patients with AIDS has only belatedly been recognized. To an often dramatic extent, each of these human tragedies can be traced to our failure to practice good antibacterial medicine. This failure is all the more painful since it has ruined the effectiveness of many of the first, true generation of Miracle Drugs, the antibiotics.

That isn't to say that researchers have remained oblivious to the dilemmas caused by the tremendous over-reliance on antibiotics. Indeed, some have been effective in alerting their national governments to the magnitude of the public health problem caused by the emergence of resistant organisms. Countries like Spain, Finland, East Germany and Turkey have had dramatic successes in reducing the amount of certain antibiotics used to treat infections, and have experienced a comparable decline in the incidence of antibiotic resistance in bacteria that cause human disease.

But even as these paltry instances of success provide proof of the ancient Chinese dictum to treat powerful medicines as if they were the arbiters of life and death, the profligate use of antibiotics has elsewhere continued unabated. In 1988, we can see the battle lines forming between physicians who are unwilling to relinquish their autonomy and clinical discretion to treat individual patients, and public health experts who want to ensure uniformity in policies that influence where and how much of a given antibiotic is used.

FOOLING MOTHER NATURE

Finland has been an epicenter of this medical morality play, where physicians bent on freely using new antibiotics for reducing the ravages of infection in their patients clashed with government policy to protect the common good by restricting their use. The drug in question is the now common antibiotic containing trimethoprim and sulfonamide, known by its brand names as Bactrim and Septra. This combination treatment was designed expressly to "outsmart" bacteria that might divise resistance to either antibiotic alone.

It was first introduced in Finland in 1969 as a means to control otherwise untreatable urinary tract infections (UTIs) that were then (as now) disrupting the lives of a significant number of adult women in developed countries around the world. Probably most of the women reading this book have experienced such infections, known commonly as "cystitis" or bladder infections, or their dangerous sequelae, kidney infection ("pyelonephritis"). To these persons, the advent of a possible cure for what is commonly an unending story of recurrent infection would be a godsend. Instead, the over-reliance (and probably misuse) of this drug spelled only a short-lived victory.

The story started familiarly enough. By 1970, only 176 kilograms of this antibiotic had been used. Thirteen years later, the annual usage in Finland alone was 2,000 kilograms and rising. At the same time, the first ominous warnings appeared that all was not well. Resistance to this "unstoppable" antibiotic was rising precipitously.

By 1984, resistance of the most common causative agent for UTIs, the common intestinal bacterium, *Escherechia coli* (or *E. coli* for short) had become the rule, not the exception in women with urinary tract infections. The insidiousness of this trend was pointed out by the finding the same year that fully 1/3 of newly hospitalized patients in nearby Sweden showed up with antibiotic resistant infections — even though none of them had been treated with this wonder drug! Similarly unanticipated resistance to trimethoprim, the major ingredient of this drug, appeared elsewhere. In the summer of 1988, children in day care centers in Houston, Texas who had never been treated with trimethoprim were found to be colonized with highly resistant bacteria.

The significance of these technical–sounding data is startling: the normal flora of our intestinal tracts can readily pick up antibiotic resistant populations — in hospital wards in Sweden, and in large day care centers in Houston. Closer investigation of the hospitals in Finland with the highest proportion of antibiotic resistance showed not only that they had overprescribed the combination antibiotic, but that many other citizens in the community had used trimethoprim to treat pets and cattle. The governments of both Scandinavian countries wanted to take action. Only Sweden outlawed the farm and non–veterinary use of these antibiotics. Finland — and the United States — continue to suffer from the dilemma of allowing veterinary and physician discretion for virtually all antibiotic use, while the public health threat from antibiotic resistant bacteria increases daily.

We now know that thousands of people in the United States have gotten *Salmonella* infections from farms that have misused antibiotics. In November, 1987, *The New England Journal of Medicine* published the most dramatic study to date showing the complicity of poor antibiotic practices in human epidemic disease. At least 675 people in Southern California developed serious antibiotic–resistant *Salmonella* infections after exposure to contaminated beef or hamburger taken from slaughtered dairy cattle. This is neither an isolated instance, nor likely to remain a limited problem as long as ignorance shapes our national policies. Unlike Sweden, up to 90 percent of all antibiotics used in agriculture here are not controlled through veterinarians. The crisis of human contamination from infected meat, carcasses and milk with antibiotic–resistant bacteria will remain a major threat until more rational national policies are adopted, a view urged in the first edition of this book.

FAILURES OF MEDICAL CONTROL

The medical community's responsibility in the emergence of drug–resistant bacteria is exemplified by gonnorhea. Here, our failure to recognize alternatives to reliance on antibiotics blind prescribing practices and patient compliance has led to an explosive epidemic. If left untreated, gonorrhea can lead to serious pelvic infection in women, and urinary and kidney infections in both men and women. Insufficient dosages and duration of therapy is known to increase the likelihood of relapse—and selection for antibiotic–resistant gonococci. Nonetheless, penicillin combined with a medication that delays its excretion continues to be prescribed in sub-optimal amounts even as the threat of wholesale antibiotic resistance grows.

In the two years since the 2nd Edition was published, there has been a 60 percent increase in the number of penicillin–resistant *Neisseria gonorrhoeae*. As a result, more and more physicians have shifted to reliance on a single (often inadequate) dose of tetracycline. By 1985, Georgia, Pennsylvania and New Hampshire all had reported cases of tetracycline resistance. The quick introduction of spectinomycin as a fall–back antibiotic to cover for this disastrous consequence met a similar fate: by May and June of 1988, the first nine cases of spectinomycin resistant gonorrhea had already appeared.

The Chicago Health Department considers the problem so serious that they issued an alert to treat *all* cases of gonorrhea with a "third generation" cephalosporin antibiotic called ceftriaxone.

This "new" (and expensive) therapeutic fix to a social problem may yet meet a similar fate. Unless antibiotic uses are coupled with sound health education about the *hygienic* measures needed to control this epidemic, no success in abating this epidemic is likely. Just such a success has been charted in the gay community, where the widespread practice of "safe sex" has led to an abatement of both AIDS *and* gonorrhea in California.

Since the last edition of this book, another organism in the same family as the gonorrhea causing bacterium has also shown up with unexpected antibiotic resistance. This time it is no plaything. It is *Neisseria meningitidis*, the organism that causes most cases of meningitis, an often fatal infection of the membrane of the brain. The antibiotic that it has shown newfound resistance to is not coincidentally also tetracycline—an essential antibacterial that had replaced much more toxic antibiotics like chloramphenicol for treating meningitis.

While the link between improperly treated gonococcal Neisseria and fatal infection with tetracycline-resistant meningococcal Neisseria remains unproven, the association appears too close to have been a chance occurrence. Clinicians now face the daunting prospect of having to treat many children with meningitis with chloramphenicol, an antibiotic that can cause fatal aplastic anemia, or find less toxic substitutes.

Clearly, we all would have been better off it more rational policies had been followed in prescribing tetracycline in the first place. These might well have included proscribing its use for treating acne, and reserving it solely for serious infections that warranted chemoprotection.

In as yet unknown ways, our antibiotic practices may be responsible for changing trends in still other bacterial scourges. The streptococcus responsible for rheumatic fever has staged a comeback, causing an epidemic of this heart-valve damaging disease in Salt Lake City in 1988. The pneumococci have had their day as well, overcoming their arch rival antibiotic, penicillin, in increasing numbers.

The response to these medical disasters has too often relied on more ingenious antibiotic combinations (e.g., new ones that mix a "bodyguard" chemical with the parent compound). More of the same is clearly not the answer. A pneumococcal vaccine, strongly advocated in my first edition, is now belatedly recognized by the World Health Organization as a long overdue—and much more rational—defense against pneumonia than is further dependence on the penicillins. Reliance on the body's own defense systems, many of which can be strengthened by diet (e.g., vitamin A or beta carotene-containing foods) or immunologic stimulants (e.g., vaccines), will prove in the end to be better solutions to most infectious diseases than are our chemical fixes.

Tuberculosis is a case in point. Thought to be a scourge confined to the ghettos and slums of yesteryear through the widespread use of BCG and related vaccines, TB has staged a resurgence. With the abatement of vaccination programs and public health complacency in detection and contact tracing, this highly infectious disease has emerged as a real killer. It now strikes a growing percentage of patients with AIDS—and increasingly, numbers of migrant farm workers and poor in the inner cities of the U.S.

Physicians presently rely on isoniazide as both a treating antibiotic and a protective one, being used "prophylactically" (i.e., for protection of those not yet diseased) to treat family members who have been in contact with a TB patient. Given the widespread reliance on this single antibiotic, it is not surprising that the TB organism has emerged in the last two years with isoniazide resistance.

Now we rely on a substitute antibiotic, rifampin for the prophylactic treatment of TB-exposed family members. But in Oregon, the wife of an isonizide resistant TB patient treated this way subsequently developed TB. It proved resistant to *both* isoniazide and rifampin! Is TB likely to stage a resurgence? The current trend of resistant organisms is a distressing index that this might happen.

In New York, 23 percent of the TB strains isolated from infected children from 1962 to 1982 were resistant to one or more of these antituberculosis drugs. The recent death of a child in New York City—during an era when TB was thought to have been eradicated—

was clearly preventable. He had been given inadequate and inappropriate treatment. In fact, his strain of TB was found to be resistant to the drugs used to treat him only after he died.

GETTING SICK IN THE HOSPITAL

In the first edition of this book, I discussed the prevalence and seriousness of infections that were acquired within the hospital. The very idea that one might get sick in a hospital is an oxymoron—hospitals are supposed to be the cleanest environments. Yet, as many as 1 in 10 in some institutions, and an average of from 2–4 percent of all hospitalized patients acquire a "nosocomial" infection from their stay. In the last several years, concern has focused one one of the more lethal forms of nosocomial infection, on that causes the progressive destruction of the lining of the intestine. In this case, the offending organism appears as a normally benign "commensal" (from the Latin phrase meaning "feeding at the same table"), living harmlessly in an average of 2–3 percent of the population's intestinal tract. In hospitalized patients, the percentage rises to 10–20 percent. The organism in question, known as *Clostridium difficile* (*C. difficile*), is in the same family as the bacterium that causes fatal food poisoning, the *botulinum* clostridium. Not surprisingly, both produce a highly poisonous toxin that causes most of the damage.

In 1988, I was an expert witness at the trial of a physician who treated a victim of these organisms and a drug company who made the broad spectrum antibiotics that set the stage for their emergence. I testified for the woman who almost died of the complications of the resulting disease known as pseudomembranous colitis. While the drug company settled the suit out of court, the physician was exonerated on the grounds that the near-fatal infection which erupted after three years and literally hundreds of courses of various ineffective antibiotic treatments was a "predictable and acceptable" risk of taking antibiotics!

During the trial, the defense attorney argued that pseudomembranous colitis was a virtually unheard of complication, so rare that no physician need warn his patients. Not so. This disease is now known to have been responsible for dozens of cases of unexplained deaths in geriatric wards—and nursing homes—where debilitated elderly patients often spend the last, tragic years of their lives. What appears to have happened in most of these cases is that the patients and fellow residents received tens of courses of broad spectrum antibiotics for often trivial or threatened infections. The result: antibiotic treatments that kill bad and good bacteria alike. After the chemical haze of battle has receded, one of the predictable survivors is the *Clostridium* species. Thriving in often new-found wastelands, the clostridia overgrow the intestinal tract of these often weakened patients, releasing vast amounts of toxins in the process.

In the hospital or nursing home, once a patient has a clostridium infection, he or she becomes an unwitting carrier that can spread the disease-causing germ to others. When it occurs in a hospital, the consequences are so extreme that the hospital's solution is often of necessity draconian. In the case of Cook County Hospital in Chicago, it meant closing an entire ward. While some antibiotics (e.g., vancomycin) can be used to treat pseudomembranous colitis, it reoccurs in almost a quarter of patients. This relapse rate ensures that a substantial number of patients remain hospitalized—and a source of infection for their ward mates. Less well appreciated is the fact that even after the closure of a ward—in one instance in England, for over three months—the clostridia can survive and remain for reinfection once a ward is reopened. "Hardy little buggers" indeed!

This hardiness—and the ease of patient to patient transmission, has led some hospitals to adopt policies that themselves create still more problems of antibiotic resistance. At Cook County Hospital, as soon as one patient develops a clostridium infection, all patients on the ward are given the antibiotics that would normally be reserved for treating only the full-blown disease.

NEW POLICY INITIATIVES

At least two antibiotics (lincomycin and clindamycin) are so commonly associated with the emergence of clostridia and the resulting pseudomembranous colitis that it is hard to justify their continued use at all. Their risk profiles for producing pseudomembranous colitis are almost 70 times that of simple penicillins, while cephalosporins carry about a 40 fold risk compared to ampicillin.

One example highlights the cascade of problems that comes from failing to recognize those risk patterns coupled with inappropriate antibiotic use. As emphasized in this book, antibiotics are rarely justified for pre-treatment of as yet uninfected patients. This so-called "prophylactic" use of antibiotics carries the risk of selecting for organisms—like the clostridia—that are hidden among the legions of normal flora in the body. At the University of Chicago hospital, researchers found that all of the women who developed clostridial infections after undergoing cesarean birth had been given a cephalosporin (cefoxitin) before the operation. None of the women who were not "prophylaxed," or who received other, less potent antibiotics, developed the disease. Nonetheless, the 1988 edition of the Merck, Sharpe and Dome volume entitled *Guide to Antimicrobial Therapy* lists cefoxitin as a drug of choice for prophylaxis during cesarean section and hysterectomy.

At stake in much of this debate is the question of how much to honor the discretionary judgment of professionals in general and physicians particularly, in choosing antibiotic regimes that may have murderous consequences for the next patient who comes along to the ward. This form of ethics, one that I call "communitarian ethics", has received scant attention in the professional literature. Instead, clinical choices appear to rely on the balance between physicians' respect for patient autonomy (weak at best), and the professional "discretion" of physicians to choose antibiotics with which they are most familiar. Such discretionary judgment often leads to disastrous consequences for an entire ward—or in the instance of the overreliance on penicillins and failure to accurately prescribe their duration and dose, the emergence of antibiotic resistant organisms that threaten whole populations.

PRESCRIBING HABITS

The starry–eyed view taken by some new physicians that antibiotics are life safers in almost any instance where a patient has a fever of unknown origin is as typical of today's practitioners as it was 10 years ago when the book first appeared. Until recently, most physicians prescribed antibiotics for "occult" or hidden bacteriemia in feverish children on the hunch (and the evidence of a few, poorly done retrospective studies) that they were heading off a potentially fatal occurrence. In a courageous (and forwardlooking) article published in *The New England Journal of Medicine* in November, 1987, researchers at Northwestern University in Chicago and children's hospitals in Philadelphia and Chicago, showed that without an idea of where an infection is coming from, antibiotics are of *no* value and may actually cause harm (by increasing the likelihood of diarrhea) in febrile, young children from 3–36 months old.

The choice to give an antibiotic "anyway" to any child with a fever is nonetheless one that is retained by many practicing pediatricians on the grounds that their clinical judgment and discretion alone dictates prescribing policy. Physician preference is a weak excuse for dangerous prescribing habits. The hazards of giving primacy to physicians who practice defensive medicine are underscored by the previously cited example in which *C. difficile* infections flared up after prophylactic use of antibiotics in women who face cesarean operations. It is well known that *if* prophylaxis is indicated surgically, a single course of antibiotics is all that is necessary. Any more, and the risk of clostridial overgrowth increases proportionately. In one outbreak of *C. difficile* among new mothers who had received "C" sections, only one third of patients received the proper *single* course of treatment. The remaining two thirds received five to ten courses of treatment. Given the questionable therapeutic value of prophylactically prescribing antibiotics in every cesarean section anyhow, the overtreatment indicated by these data comes close to professional irresponsibility.

Dentists are among the worst offenders in relying too much on the "pre-emptive strike" philosophy of protection against infection. Under this maxim, the clinician relies on a kind of shot-gun effect conferred by a blind dose of a broad-spectrum (affecting many different kinds of bacteria) antibiotic given before and after an invasive procedure. In oral surgery, antibiotics given for one week were compared with giving antibiotics of three *months* (in the absence of evidence of active infection) after root canal or gum surgery. *Neither* regimen proved better than withholding antibiotics altogether. Yet the author of the study concluded that one week was best.

Many of the problems resulting from over-reliance on antibiotics can be obviated by strict adherence to published guidelines for using special tests of suspected bacteria to establish their sensitivity to a given antibiotic *before* that antibiotic is used. Culture and sensitivity testing provide a critical link from the microbe to an appropriate medication. They are as often omitted as included in contemporary charts, in spite of written hospital management and drug surveillance management orders which mandate their use.

A recent study of antibiotic request forms provides a typical example: the most common omission was the rationale for choosing the drug requested! Without a clear understanding of the indications and limitations of proposed therapeutic agents (to say nothing of side-effects), little long-term success may be expected in devising rational strategies that ultimately increase rather than decrease the effectiveness of antibiotics.

All too often, these seemingly expensive sensitivity tests (expensive in the short run) are averted by substituting a good guess, "empiric" therapy. The choice of a hot, new antibiotic is expected to get results, often because its very newness reduces the statistical likelihood that resistant bacteria exist in sufficient numbers to thwart the therapy. Yet, it is precisely this shot-gunning technique that ultimately shortens the effective lifespan of that antibiotic, since blind use is a sure fire way to select for resistant germs. For drug companies that thrive on selling a lot of products, such a practice virtally assures the demand for a "new model" in the near future. Only in those countries that have adopted conservative antibiotic regimes (which appears to be happening in Spain currently), do the old mainstays of effective chemotherapy like penicillin, ampicillin and erythromycin stand a chance of remaining in the effective pharmacopaeia.

A little known fact about sensitivity testing is that once "empiric" (literally, experimental) therapy is begun, it is often difficult to find enough of the offending bacteria to run an adequate test. This reality belies the urging of drug company advertisements to commence sensitivity testing as soon as possible *after* emergency start-up of empiric therapy. There is a therapeutic blind spot that is hidden by the seeming rationale for instituting therapy on the first visit (an outcome often demanded by the patient). What may appear to be the expedient and necessary first course of treatment, may prove wrong on reexamination of cultures (if successful) taken later on. Moreover, the consequences of a failed course of antibiotic therapy should the infecting organism prove resistant to the "best-guess" antibiotic, are often much more dire and expensive than instituting a policy of routine testing of every patient.

The ramifications for the patient are obvious—an infection that doesn't go away. But the consequences for the population as a whole—which are often the tragic cost of professional discretion and diagnostic short cuts—remain little appreciated. As long as drug-resistant bacteria go unchecked, their opportunity to spread and increase throughout the community continues. No one truly knows the consequences of exposing millions of other bacteria to an array of antibiotics intended for unrelated villains. Certainly, one of those consequences is the seemingly "benign" emergence of anti-biotic resistant bacteria among our native, and sometimes essential, microbial denizens. Antibiotic resistant intestinal bacteria—our friend, *E. coli*—may be benign, but if they acquire certain genes they can be converted into fatal offenders, causing enterotoxigenic shock and incurable urinary tract infections.

ALTERNATIVES

The linked ecological arguments advanced in this book—that we need to limit antibiotic use to prevent spread of intractable infections, and to strengthen alternative forms of therapy—are based on the belief that with pharmaceuticals as with much else, less is more. How much attention have we lavished on developing new drugs at the expense of recognizing the need to maximize the natural defenses inherent in our immune systems, or the simple expedients of public health hygiene?

Among the alternatives that were advocated in the first edition of the book, vaccines remain the most undervalued and potentially most far reaching interventions available to circumvent the never-ending cycle of drugs and antibiotic resistance. While antibiotics will always have a place in our armamentarium against infectious disease (if sparingly, and rationally used), vaccines can be developed only by the concerted will and effort of the federal government.

As much as we overuse the technological solutions seemingly conferred by antibiotics, we have grossly underused the technological advances that have long been on the shelf for making vaccines against bacterial and viral targets. Unlike the notorious influenza virus which is constantly evolving, novel antigenic types that elude the immune system, most bacteria are relatively homogenous, and offer relatively easy targets for an activated immune system. The long-awaited vaccine against Pseudomonas infection, a common cause of serious bacterial sepsis in burn victims, appears little closer to reality than when it was first called for in my first edition. We have to ask, then, why more effort has not gone into vaccine development. One simplistic answer is that such development is seen as a high-risk enterprise by most drug companies concerned about "sure-thing" profitability. For many, the idea of vaccine development is replete with legal pitfalls, as well as more understandable technical difficulties of correctly identifying and packaging the proper bacterial, parasitic or viral antigens.

Presently, many drug companies perceive vaccine development to be fraught with problems of liability. Many drug companies believe they are in jeopardy—and without insurance—if they attempt manufacture and testing without adequate safeguards. A federal program to safeguard and underwrite innovative drug companies is long overdue. Many vaccines are available for use today, but are going begging for want of adequate assurance that a company marketing them will be exempt from liability. Congress has recently taken a step in the right direction by enacting legislation intended to indemnify manufacturers, but full protection is still wanting.

In the meantime, vaccines targeted at high risk groups are receiving sparse, but needed attention. In 1985, a vaccine against the most common cause of middle ear infections and meningitis in children, *Hemophilus influenzae* type B was finally marketed, after years of frustrating delay. The particular virtue of this vaccine is that it would greatly reduce the undue reliance on antibiotics that presently characterizes pediatric care and prophylaxis of middle ear infection with effusion and meningitis. For public health reasons alone, the National Advisory Committee on Immunization for Canada and its American counterpart both recommend that all children receive this vaccine once they have reached two years (below that age, the immunization process is less effective).

Some centers appear to be using the vaccine, but only under circumstances that contradict the basic public health protection rationale indicated by this endorsement. Studies of day care children clearly show that the vaccine was the most effective (on the basis of cost *and* benefit) in protecting classmates of victims of *H. influenzae* infections. Why *all* the children in day care centers are not immunized against this potentially deadly bacterium is difficult to fathom—until one recognizes the depth of the lack of support for vaccination in the United States.

As an example, community and Health Department clinics surveyed in Texas were found to have administered the vaccine only about 10 percent of the occasions when its use was indicated. A portion of the blame for this shameful statistic is that the majority of clinics received no state or federal dollars to administer the vaccine.

Similar tales of woeful support for the concept of vaccination can be found elsewhere. In spite of a March, 1988 recommendation to the World Health Organization, members of the European community still do not routinely recommend pneumococcal vaccination for the elderly. In Europe, as well as some states like Illinois in the United States, a substantial portion of the adults in the community are also unprotected against diptheria and tetanus. In Denmark, a quarter of the adult population is unvaccinated against diptheria. Still higher numbers can be found in Sweden (50–70 percent); England (33–41 percent); and West Germany (68 percent). These data not only mean that the stage is set for major epidemics of highly transmissable disease, but that the concommitant reliance on antibiotic use for its treatment is undobutedly going to increase in these countries.

In the United States, protection against debilitating diseases among the elderly is still incomplete and, in many instances, ineffectual. While the poor success rate for combatting influenza is well known (on average only 1 in 5 are immunized in any given year), the wide, mandated availability of a pneumococcal vaccine has not led to any greater use. Only 10 percent of elderly patients entering the emergency room of a major U.S. hospital had ever received the potentially life saving pneumococcal vaccine. In view of the higher mortality of pneumonia in victims who carry antibiotic resistant infections (in one study 54 percent versus 25 percent), often from previous antibiotic treatments, the continued reliance on a chemical rather than an immunologic venue to protection appears irrational.

The simple truth is that while we continue to reinforce the burgeoning antibiotic industry, we lack any systematic approach to immunization in this country. This omission is particularly tragic when it comes to AIDS.

Many AIDS victims would have benefitted from pre-HIV infection immunization with even a minimum of the standard vaccines. Even after they are ill, immunization against opportunisitc organisms can prove beneficial. Unexpectedly, patients with AIDS can get much needed benefits from vaccination against pneumococci and *H. influenzae.* Since these are two major causes of infection that antibiotics can only partially subdue in AIDS patients, the discovery that HIV positive men can mount an immune response following immunization with these vaccines opens up a previously underappreciated line of defense against the opportunistic infections that most commonly cause their death.

All of this underscores the failure of public health education in both the lay and professional communities of the essential role of immunizations in this country. The lack of readiness of the public to accept and the medical community to deliver proven vaccines is a tragic example. The Hepatitis B vaccine, which was introduced in 1982, was supposed to be used by everyone in high risk groups— workers who are exposed to blood, staff and clients of institutions for the developmentally disabled, and the workers in hemodialysis units. Up to 30 percent of such persons can develop the debilitating liver disease caused by hepatitis B. But today, fewer than half of the persons in any one of these groups has been vaccinated.

Instead of decreasing following the advent of an effective vaccine (as has been the pattern in the past), Hepatitis B has increased over 25 percent since the vaccine was introduced (from 9.2/100,000 persons in 1981 to 11.5/100,000 in 1986). The biggest increase mirrors the disastrous epidemiology of the AIDS epidemic: fully 28 percent of intravenous drug abusers were infected by the Hepatitis B virus in 1987, up from 15 percent just five years earlier.

Part of the problem is a draconian public health system which requires, in almost 1/4 of the health settings studied, that the workers pay for their own vaccinations, and limits access of IV drug abusers to a health system which they fear rather than trust.

WHAT THE DOCTOR CAN DO

Health workers themselves harbor irrational fears about vaccines. Studies of their attitudes reveal that many—sometimes a majority— of health workers in high risk professions deny that proven vaccines are safe or effective for them to use. Over time, health professionals in the highest risk groups for acquiring hepatitis develop unsound perceptions of their own invincibility, believing (erroneously) that they are robust and less susceptible to infection that their normal counterparts.

This therapeutic blind spot is reflected in the dismal success of hospitals, governmental agencies and clinics to get the medical professions to comply with even simple hand-washing procedures.

Since the days of Semmelweis in the 19th century, it has been axiomatic that reduction in bacterial or other transmissable diseases begins at the sink. (Semmelweiss was the first to show that peurperal fever, which occurred commonly after assisted childbirth, could be drastically reduced by mid-wives and physicians washing *before* rather than after delivery).

The simple expedient of wearing a protective gown, washing hands thoroughly, and avoiding touching one's *own* body or orifices (the nose is a prime offender) has been shown in study after study to do more to reduce inter-patient infections than any other single procedure or chemical solution.

The medical professional's sense of invulnerability coupled with naturophobia (distaste for biological products) in favor of chemical ones points to a terrible weak point in our collective mentality. We continue to believe—erroneously—that the microbial world will submit to our chemical ministrations and behave in an orderly and predictable manner. Time after time, our conservative expectations (*no* bacterium was supposed to be found that was resistant to 8 antibiotics, combination antibiotics would solve the resistance problems, etc., etc.) have been dashed. Clearly a new ethic is needed if we are to successfully integrate our lives with those of the microbial world.

OUR IMMUNE SYSTEM
AND THE GLOBAL ECOSYSTEM

The final arbiter of success or failure in fighting infection is our immune system. Chemicals, such as the dioxins and furans which can decimate this system (as can other ubiquitous environmental chemicals such as PCBs), are daily realities of our lives. If we do not protect and nurture an effective and healthly immune system, we are at great peril. The recent die off of harbor seals in Sweden, affecting almost 1/3 of the population, echoes similar decimating infectious diseases that have wiped out shore-line populations of oceanic mammals in North America. Both are probably due to toxic chemical immunosuppression.

In the end, the major insight which the antibiotic saga has provided is the recognition that the bacterial ecosystem with which we co-exist is a genetically continuous, global population. Just as in weather theory it can be said that a butterfly flapping its wings in Brazil can cause a tornado in Kansas, even seemingly inconsequential events such as the emergence of a single case of antibiotic resistant pneumococci in South Africa can lead to global catastrophe as drug resistance spreads throughout the world.

We can no longer think of patients with serious infections as if they were isolated individuals. Once treated inappropriately, the individual harboring drug resistant bacteria poses a threat to his spouse, neighbor, ward–mate and ultimately the entire population. The contemporary naivete that simply because only a small porportion of bacteria are likely to emerge resistant from any one course of therapy gives a green light to "empiric" treatment, is setting the stage for still greater public health disasters.

No man is an island in the universe of microorganisms. We are all interconnected. A mistake made in one corner of the world ultimately will come full circle to haunt us. With the growing, albeit grudging acceptance of our global interrelatedness, this is an opportune moment to stop and reflect how our well-intentioned efforts at self-protection with overuse of antibiotics put others at risk.

It is time for a new ethic for medicine generally, one that recognizes this interrelatedness. What better place to start than in the ongoing saga of the conflict with the microbial world. As with the Soviet Union, what is needed is a recognition that we create our own security by recognizing our interdependence. Peristroika in the microbial world may mean that we have to readjust our chemical dependence and look for more harmonious solutions to the problem of germs that won't die.

University of Illinois
College of Medicine
August 1988

*The research assistance of Kimberly Warner, D Pharm in gathering materials for this Preface is gratefully acknowledged.

BIBLIOGRAPHY

Akalin, H. Erdel, Torum, Mustafa and Alacam, Ruhi. "Amino-glycoside resistance patterns in Turkey," *Scandinavian Journal of Infectious Disease* 20: 199–203, 1988.

Anonymous. "Hepatitis B rise noted among drug abusers," *Chicago Tribune*, July 22, 1988, Sec 1. page 5.

Anonymous. "Recommendations of the Immunization Practices Advisory Committee: Update on Hepatitis B Prevention," *Morbidity and Mortality Weekly Report* 36: 437–449, 1987.

Anonymous. "Survey of parents' attitudes to the recommended *Haemophilus influenzae* type b vaccine program;" *Canadian Medical Association Journal* 137: 371, 1987.

Aronsson, B. Mollby, R. and Nord, C. E. "Antimicrobial agents and *Clostridium difficile* in acute enteric disease: Epidemiological data from Sweden, 1980–1982," *Journal of Infectious Diseases* 151: 476–481, 1985.

Arsura, Edward L., Fazio, Richard A. and Wickremesinghe, Prasanna C. "Pseudomonas colitis following prophylactic antibiotic use in primary cesarean section," *American Journal of Obstetrics and Gynecology* 151: 87–89, 1985.

Block, Barry S., Mercer, Lane J., Ismail, Mahmoud A. and Moawad, Atef H. "*Clostridium difficile*-associated diarrhea follows perioperative prophylaxis with cefoxitin," *American Journal of Obstetrics and Gynecology* 153: 835–838, 1985.

Brahams, Diana. "Damages for stroke after cholera and typhoid vaccination," *The Lancet* ii: 1372, 1985.

Brewer Ford, Matuszak, Diane I., Libonati Joseph P. et al. "Tetracycline resistant Neisseria," *New England Journal of Medicine* 315: 1548–1549, 1986.

Broome, Claire V., Mortimer, Edward A., Katz, Samuel L. et al, "Special Report: Use of chemoprophylaxis to prevent the spread of *Hemophilus influenzae* B in day-care facilities," *New England Journal of Medicine* 316: 1227–1228, 1987.

Caison, C. "*Neisseria gonorrhoeae:* a versatile pathogen," *J Clin Pathol* 40: 1088–1097, 1987.

Carter, Anne O., Borczyk, Alexander A., Carlson, Jacqueline A. K., et al. "A severe outbreak of *Escherichia coli* 0157:H7-associated hemorragic colitis in a nursing home," *New England Journal of Medicine* 317: 1496–1500, 1987.

Chwatt-Bruce, L. J. "Recent trends of chemotherapy and vaccination against malaria: New lamps for old," *British Medical Journal* 291: 1072–1076, 1985.

Crumplin, G. C. "Plasmid-mediated resistance to nalidixic acid and new 4-quinolones?," *The Lancet* ii: 854–855, 1987.

Cryz, S. J., Sadoff, J. C. and Furer, E. "Immunization with a *Pseudomonas aeruginosa* immunotype 50 polysaccharide-toxin A conjugate vaccine: Effect of a booster dose on antibody levels in humans," *Infection and Immunity* 6: 1829–1830, 1988.

Faller, Michale A., Wakefield, Douglas S., Hammons, G. T. et al. "Variation from standards in *Staphylococcus aureus* susceptibility testing," *American Journal of Clinical Pathology* 88: 231–235, 1987.

Fedson, David S. "Penicillin-resistant pneumococci," *The Lancet* ii: 1451–1452, 1988 (letter).

Fulton, John P., Bodenheimer, Henry C., and Kramer, Peter D. "Acceptance of Hepatitis B vaccine among hospital workers: A follow-up," *American Journal of Public Health* 76: 1339–1340, 1986.

Goldman, Donald A. and Klinger, Jeffrey D. "*Pseudomonas cepacia:* Biology, mechanisms of virulence, epidemiology, "*Journal of Pediatrics* 108: 806–812, 1986.

Goldstein F. W., Chumpitaz, J. C., Guevara, G. M., et al. "Plasmid-mediated resistance to multiple antibiotics in *Salmonella typhi,*" *Journal of Infectious Diseases* 153: 261–266, 1986.

Gould, F. K., Magee, J. G. and Ingham, H. R. "A hospital outbreak of antibiotic resistant *Streptococcus pneumoniae,*" *Journal of Infection* 15: 77–79, 1987.

Gururaj, Vymutt J., Patrick, Jenny K. and Fields-Rogers, Patricia. "*Haemophilus influenzae* Type b vaccine: Use in the pediatric population," *Pediatrics* 80: 731–735, 1987.

Hay, Joel W. and Daum, Robert S. "Cost-benefit analysis of two strategies for prevention of *Haemophilus influenzae* Type b infection," *Pediatrics* 80: 319–329, 1987.

Hemsell, David L., Hemsell, Patricia G., Healrd, Molly L., et al. "Preoperative cefoxitin prophylaxis for elective abdomnal hysterectomy;" *American Journal of Obstetrics and Gynecology* 153: 255–226, 1985.

Hooper, David C., Wolfson, John S., Ng, Eva Y et al. "Mechanisms of action and resistance to ciprofloxacin," *American Journal of Medicine* 82: 12–20, 1987.

Huang, Juo-Liang, Ruben, Frederick L., Rnaldo, Charles R., et al. "Antibody responses after influenza and pneumococcal immunization in HIV-infected homosexual men," *Journal of the American Medical Association* 257: 2047–2050, 1987.

Jaffe, David M., Tanz, Robert R., Davis, Todd et al. "Antibiotic administration to treat possible occult bacteremia in febrile children," *New England Journal of Medicine* 317: 1175–1180, 1987.

Kjeldsen, Keld, Simonsen, Ole and Heron, Iver. "Immunity against diptheria and tetanus in the age group 30–70 years," *Scandinavian Journal of Infectious Disease* 20: 177–185, 1988.

Larson, Elaine, "A causal link between handwashing and risk of infection. Examination of the evidence," *Infection Control and Hospital Epidemiology* 9: 28–36, 1988.

Livengood, John R., Sigler, Judi G., Foster, Laurence R. et al. "Isoniazid-resistant tuberculosis," *Journal of the American Medical Association* 253: 2847–2849, 1985.

Neu, Harold C. "New antibiotics: Areas of appropriate use," *Journal of Infectious Diseases* 155: 403–417, 1987.

Olson, Bruce, Weinstein, Robert A., Nathan, Catherine, et al. "Occult aminoglycoside resistance in *Pseudomonas aeruginosa:* Epidemiology and implications for therapy and control," *Journal of Infectious Diseases* 151: 769–774, 1985.

Pallares, R. "Pneumococcal disease: A change in antibiotic susceptibility and therapy, "*APUA Newsletter* 6: 7, 1988.

Pallares, Roman, Gudiol, Francisco, Linares Josefina et al. "Risk factors and response to antibiotic therapy in adults with bacteremic pneumonia caused by penicillin-resistant pneumococci," *New England Journal of Medicine* 317: 18–19, 1987.

Polish, Michael A., Smith Jeffrey P., Sainer, Deborah et al. "Prospects for an emergency department-based adult immunization program," *Archives of Internal Medicine* 147: 1919–2001, 1987.

Ranta, Helena, Haapusalo, Markus and Ranta, Kari et al, "Bacteriology of odontogenic apical periodontitis and effect of penicillin treatment," *Scandinavian Journal of Infectious Disease* 20: 187–192, 1988.

Rao, Salini, Jacobs, Sharn and Joyce, Linda. "Cost effective eradication of an outbreak of methicillin-resistant *Staphylococcus aureus* in a community teaching hospital," *Infection Control and Hospital Epidemiology* 9: 255–260, 1988.

Reves, RR, and Barbara E Murray. "Trimethoprim–resistant *E. coli* among children in day care centers in Houston," *APUA Newsletter* 6: 1–2, 1988.

Sander, Christine C. "Emergence of resistance to B-lactams, aminoglycosides, and quinolones during combination therapy for infection due to *Serratia marcescens,*" *Journal of Infectious Diseases* 153: 617–619, 1986.

Schwalbe, Richard S., Stapleton, Jack T. and Gilligan, Peter H., "Emergence of vancomycin resistance in coagulase-negative staphylococci," *New England Journal of Medicine* 316: 927–931, 1987.

Spika, Hohn S., Waterman, Stephen H. and Soo Hoo, G. W., et al. "Chloramphenicol-resistant *Salmonella newport* traced through hamburger to diary farms—A Major persisting source of human salmonellosis in California," *New England Journal of Medicine* 316: 565–570, 1987. (See also Letters in *NEJM* 317: 632, 3 September 1987).

Steiner, Phillip, Rao, Madu Mao, Mitchell, Millicent, et al. "Primary drug-resistant tuberculosis in children," *American Journal of Diseases of Children* 13: 780–782, 1985.

Talbot, R. W., Walker, R. C. and Beart R. W. Jr. "Changing epidemiology, diagnosis, and treatment of *Clostridium difficile* toxin-associated colitis," *Journal of Surgery* 73: 457–460, 1986.

Turner, A., Jephcott, A. E. and Gough, K. R. "Tetracycline-resistant meningococci," *The Lancet* ii: 1454, 1988.

Veasy, George L,., Wiedmeier, Susan E., Orsmond, Garth S., "Resurgence of acute rheumatic fever in the intermountain area of the United States, *New England Journal of Medicine* 316: 421–427, 1987.

Weisser, Jochen and Wiedemann, Bernd. "Brief report: Effects of ciprofloxacin on plasmids," *American Journal of Medicine* 82: 21–22, 1987.

When Antibiotics Fail

1

Introduction: The Medusa Effect

During the last ten years, the face of the medical world has been transformed by a silent revolution of bacterial diseases with heightened resistance to the most commonly used miracle drugs of our era: the antibiotics. Epidemics of infections caused by resistant organisms have broken out with disturbing regularity in hospitals and nurseries. In surgical and burn wards where major medical advances have permitted the survival of otherwise doomed patients, previously benign bacteria have emerged with new disease-causing activity. Suddenly, physicians throughout the world are being confronted with hitherto unrecognized or infrequently encountered infectious diseases, many of which are dangerously resistant to treatment with antibiotics.

As a result the modern-day physician must contend with an expanding and changing spectrum of infectious diseases that often appear impervious to the standard and previously effective modes of therapy. In response to this new challenge, pharmaceutical firms have redoubled their efforts to generate new antibiotics to bolster the flagging armamentarium presently in use. In the meantime, antibiotic-resistant bacteria responsible for diverse diseases of the intestinal tract, lungs, skin, and bladder are sweeping vulnerable populations of the young, old, and infirm with disturbing regularity.

Item: Between 1977 and the end of 1979, 310 cases of a new form of salmonellosis (food poisoning) are recorded in Britain. All 310 infections prove multiply resistant to antibiotics, and two persons die. Strangely, the same patterns of resistance in the causative agent appear in salmonella bacteria infecting dairy cattle.

Item: In 1979, in Middlesbrough, England, fourteen children in a nursery are infected by salmonella bacteria that prove resistant to seven different antibiotics. The attending physicians must stand by helplessly and let the infection take its course. Fortunately, all survive.

Item: A routine case of severe diarrhea is treated with penicillin and the seemingly well fifteen-month-old boy is encouraged to return to his day care group after the standard course of treatment. The bacteria causing the diarrhea survive treatment and three weeks later, eight out of ten of his playmates are ill.

Item: In 1976, a group of Vietnam veterans returning to the United States via the Philippines brings back a strain of gonorrhea that is resistant to penicillin known as "PPNG" (penicillinase-producing *Neisseria gonorrhoeae*). Five years later, PPNG has spread to major cities on both the East and West coasts. By mid-1981, it is responsible for one out of every three cases of VD reported in Los Angeles, and has been found in ninety-nine persons in Florida, an increase of 650 percent from the previous year.

Item: In 1977, a ward of children in a pediatric nursery in Durban, South Africa, develop a disturbingly hard-to-treat pneumococcal infection. For the first time in history, this normally easily controlled infection proves resistant to three unrelated, major antibiotics. In Colorado during November 1980, a seriously ill eleven-month-old infant with meningitis is discovered to harbor an identical strain of *Streptococcus pneumoniae*.

These seemingly isolated episodes are part of an interconnected series of events that add up to a worldwide picture of diseases that are increasingly resistant to the standard means of control via antibiotics. The pattern of events that emerges is strikingly consistent: a new chemotherapeutic agent is introduced and used prodigiously with little regard for the susceptibility of the organisms it was designed to attack; somewhere in the world, an organism appears that has mastered the microchemistry to resist the agent; and, in an astonishingly short period, that organism's descendants become the new enemy. In time, a new antibiotic is developed, more resistant strains appear, and the pattern of antibiotic roulette begins anew.

While epidemiologists try to grasp the full extent of this dramatic new problem, hospitals and clinics have belatedly installed surveillance procedures and often ill-conceived control measures that have barely begun to stem the tide of antibiotic-resistant infections. By conservative estimate, such infections are responsible for at least a hundred thousand deaths a year, and the toll is mounting.

The response to this devastating toll has been weak at best. Many concerned clinicians find their hands tied by the traditional mores of their colleagues who demand total freedom and discretion in prescribing practices. While countries like Japan, Czechoslovakia, and Sweden have clamped down on the free availability of antibiotics for prescription, others like Mexico, Brazil, and Guatemala permit the most potent and toxic antibiotics like chloramphenicol to be sold over-the-counter. As inappropriate or suboptimal use of any antibiotic can encourage the emergence of new resistant organisms, and as this resistance can be rapidly spread across national boundaries, one would expect such practices to be aggressively discouraged.

Instead, both in the United States and abroad, a virtual paralysis against effective action prevails. Here, antibiotics are freely given to livestock with complete disregard for the scientific advice that warns against creating still another reservoir of antibiotic-resistant organisms.

Organisms almost totally resistant to the major antibiotics now run rampant in hospital quarters, nurseries, and animal stockyards alike, creating unprecedented problems for infectious disease control specialists and public health officials. In spite of the awesome nature and speed of this spread of resistant organisms, many American agencies like the Center for Disease Control in Atlanta, Georgia, have only recently recognized the full implications of this problem. Hospitals and physicians still only grudgingly admit that a problem exists, even as new antibiotics appear to proliferate as fast as the old ones are outstripped by resistant organisms.

Chief among the forces that shaped the antibiotic revolution was the almost boundless optimism that attended the discovery of penicillin, the first "natural" antibiotics, and later, the means to synthesize the core of the penicillin molecule itself. With this second level of control came the possibility of an almost endless profusion of synthetic and semisynthetic antibiotics—and a concomitant belief that the incomplete demise of major infectious diseases that came with the introduction of antibiotics merely signaled suboptimal chemical effectiveness. A closer look at the geography and time course of the spread of epidemic, antibiotic-resistant infections could have told a different story, but American practitioners would have none of it: They had their miracle drugs.

The reasons for this blind optimism can be attributed to at least three factors: First, in the early 1940s, only a few microorganisms accounted for most of the major infectious diseases. Second, the diseases they produced, like "strep" throat, pneumonia, boils, and furuncles, were readily identified by the bedside physician. Third, and most important, these diseases were among those most susceptible to antibiotic treatments. When changing patterns of hospitalization, antibiotic treatments, hygiene, and newborn care rapidly created a new universe of infectious organisms, many physicians were simply unprepared by training and expectations to meet the challenge.

But behind this continuing struggle with prodigious microorganisms like the staphylococcus or gonococcus may lie a more basic tale: the hubris of human nature which leads us to believe that we can attain absolute control over the natural world. The development of antibiotics can be seen as an extension of the same world view which led to Paul Ehrlich's mislabeled "magic bullet" (Salvarsan) in the fight against syphilis. In our time, simplistic models of genetic change and susceptibility to antibiotics led to the naïve presumption that bacterial disease could be wiped out in our lifetime.

Somewhere along the way the miracle of natural bacterial killers became tarnished. The first exuberant reports of clinical success (sulfanilamide in 1933, penicillin in 1938) gave way to profound pessimism among some scientific observers as one strain after another appeared to be transformed into new, more resistant strains, or were replaced by totally different pathogens.

Shortly after antibiotics came into widespread use during World War II, it became clear that some germs were going to prove resistant to their lethal or growth-inhibiting effects. As early as 1942, Sir Alexander Fleming, who had discovered penicillin some thirteen years earlier, warned the medical profession about the appearance of antibiotic resistance among the staphylococci.

By that time, researchers had already discovered that bacteria contained an enzyme that could break off the molecular core of penicillin, the beta-lactam ring. Those who knew penicillin best recognized in this discovery, that they were in for a battle. The occurrence of serious clinical problems stemming from treatment failures came swiftly on the heels of laboratory bench theory. Appeals for care in using penicillin fell on deaf ears.

In 1944, just as this wonder drug appeared on the American market, Dr. Howard W. Florey, the British codeveloper (with Ernst B. Chain) and selfless entrepreneur who had brought penicillin to the United States, vainly decried the misuse that was already apparent. Florey admonished, "It is clearly futile to attempt penicillin treatment when the organism concerned is insensitive."[1]

[1] H. W. Florey, "Clinical use of penicillin," *British Medical Journal,* 2: 9–13, 1944.

He noted that some coliform organisms actually increased during a course of penicillin treatment, and warned that still other bacteria appeared whose potential for infection or harm was but barely understood. Finally, Florey prophetically warned that penicillin's effectiveness might already be waning, and cited clinical cases that had already required four to eight times the starting dose of antibiotic before control of the infection could be gained.

In spite of these lone voices, popular scientific accounts of the period from 1942 through 1958 heralded virtually every new antibiotic as part of the growing consortium of "wonder drugs" that promised to halt the few remaining infectious diseases that had been the scourge of previous civilizations. By 1955, when a few genuinely frightening diseases like scarlet fever *had* been subdued by penicillin, antibiotics had become so popular that they were being proposed as routine additives to crop sprays, food preservatives, and animal feeds. Apple, pear, walnut, and bean blights were to be wiped out with penicillin and previous repositories of lurking infection such as hamburger and chipped ice were to be sanitized with massive doses of tetracycline. So many dairy cows were being treated with antibiotics to prevent mastitis that a market survey conducted in 1955 showed that almost 12 percent of 474 milk samples from all over the country were contaminated with penicillin. Today, traces of antibiotic residues are still found in meat products, raising the prospect of low-level selection of antibiotic-resistant bacteria in healthy persons.

The short-lived but seemingly dramatic effectiveness of each new generation of antibiotics encouraged drug companies to continue their quest for modern-day versions of Ehrlich's magic bullet. But a few epidemiologists raised voices of concern about the almost mindless proliferation of uses that this glut has produced. Could the emergence of these new varieties of antibiotic-resistant bacteria be due to some of these nonmedical applications? And what about the apparent spread of resistance from one kind of bacterium to another?

We now know that the rapid spread of new microbes suddenly made resistant is in part attributable to the appearance of what is called "infectious drug resistance," a process in which microorganisms disperse parts of their genetic material from one bacterium to another. (The vehicle for this transfer is often a special DNA molecule known as an R factor.)

A second cluster of events which have contributed to the incomplete success of even the most effective of antibiotics is related to the paucity of clear thinking about national and international policies needed to employ antibiotics rationally. Many practitioners have been slow to appreciate that agricultural and economic policies for using antibiotics have ramifications which transcend national boundaries.

Beneath the apparently calm surface of diplomacy over our own antibiotic additions to animal feeds lies a global struggle championed by multinational corporations to secure their "prerogative" to grow livestock under the most economical conditions. And beneath the apparent success in annihilating diseases which plague the underdeveloped countries of the world lies a xenophobic concern for not importing them here. Malaria, gonorrhea, and tuberculosis, diseases now often resistant to the antibiotics which were first employed to control them, are now seen as threatening to our own country's public health.

Our seeming concern for the spread of human misery brought about indirectly through short-sighted policies has often proven self-serving and highly discriminatory. When an antibiotic like chloramphenicol proves so toxic that its use must be sharply curtailed in this country, there is little hesitation to export the bulk of the surplus to countries like Brazil and Mexico where it can be purchased over-the-counter like so much cough medicine—and without any warning of the dire consequence of bone marrow damage which can accompany its use.

Closer to home, you might learn that the community hospital is the most dangerous place to be if your body's defenses are weakened by malnutrition or disease. Hospital garbage and wastes—like the enormous outfalls from feedlots—are ready-made sources of contagion for antibiotic-resistant bacteria. And many hospital staff members walk around like latter-day "Typhoid Marys" (named after Mary Mallon, the New York food handler who infected at least 51 people in 1915 with typhoid fever). Many nurses and residents have been found to harbor antibiotic-resistant organisms that they acquired in the hospital. Some become chronic carriers of such microbes, bearing multiply resistant staph in their nasal passages, and *Pseudomonas* and other stubborn bacteria on their hands and skin.

Even though they are usually remarkably nontoxic, antibiotics like penicillin are potential time bombs for anyone whose immune system develops a reaction to them. Highly allergenic antibiotics are still responsible for hundreds of deaths from anaphylactic shock around the world. By the 1960s, the second generation of antibiotics were also found to have their own dangerous side effects.

More ominously, at this time, a second group of organisms began to emerge with extraordinary resistance to the wonder drugs. Gonococcus strains which were once obliterated with a hundred thousand units of penicillin began to require more than five million; new mutations began to appear that gave the ubiquitous gonococcus organism virtually total immunity to penicillins or its contemporary substitute, spectinomycin. Staph strains followed suit.

Elsewhere the story took an even more frightening turn: bacteria which were "proven" to be incapable of acquiring resistance to any more than two or three different antibiotics began to show up with resistance to six, seven, and even twelve different antibiotics. The early warnings by Japanese researchers in the mid-1950s about strange new "resistance factors" among dysentery bacteria (*Shigella*) went unnoticed or were ignored.

R factors, which permit the transfer of antibiotic resistance from one organism to another, were found to cross between totally unrelated bacteria, making the antibiotic game one of deadly roulette. If all the members of a given infecting organism were not killed outright, the few survivors who had mutations conferring resistance to that drug not only multiplied, but might also spread their defensive genes to other microorganisms. In time, even previously benign organisms, like the inhabitants of our intestinal tract (*Escherichia coli*), appeared with multiple drug resistance which could be passed on to their more virulent cousins via R factors.

Now we are faced with immensely complex policy decisions: should we use antibiotics in animal feeds to enhance cattle or poultry growth, saving cost and improving production? Or should we give priority to the health of farmers who tend these animals and through contact can pick up newly emerged resistant bacteria? Should antibiotics like clindamycin, which have extremely hazardous side effects, be left in the general pharmacopeia where a prescription by an uninformed physician can cause serious injury or death? And should new antibiotics be sought at increased consumer, as well as producer, expense which only promise to perpetuate this dangerous evolutionary cat-and-mouse game?

How should we use our primitive understanding of the massive disruption of the natural ecology of microorganisms caused by the unrestricted use of antibiotics to set new policies? Who bears the responsibility—and cost—of the sudden appearance and proliferation of these new antibiotic-resistant strains? Finally, how do we reconcile the often conflicting claims of individual physicians and their patients with those of the community at large?

Although recommendations have been made to monitor antibiotic use or to provide prescription guidelines, progress in actually reducing the emergence of resistant strains has been negligible. Our almost total passivity in the face of a medical problem of such portentous dimensions is difficult to explain and frightening in its implications. If we are to retain our toehold over the continuing menace of powerful infectious agents, it would appear to require a clean break from the patterns of the recent past.

Instead, like the ancient mortals of Greek mythology who were turned to stone by the snake-haired visage of Medusa, many public health officials and clinicians today appear petrified in the face of the transformations of the bacterial world. The response to these transformations has been to continue in the same path that we tried in the past: throw more antibiotics with more chemical nuances against the organisms that resisted the first onslaught. As with the petrified remains of fallen heroes, on the remote island where Medusa and her two Gorgon sisters lived, the battlefield of infectious diseases may soon be littered with the bodies of protagonists of the antibiotics that were used in a vain attempt to subdue the enemy by direct force.

We may wish to contemplate the success of Perseus in finally beheading the immortal Medusa and thereby quelling her threat to the world of mortals. Unlike his predecessors, Perseus attacked Medusa by looking at her obliquely in the reflection of his shield. New approaches to the problem of immortal antibiotic-resistant organisms may require similarly inventive attacks.

2

The Extent of the Problem

The true extent to which the number and severity of major epidemics of human disease have been enhanced through the proliferation of antibiotic-resistant bacteria may never be known. Where epidemiologists have charted human diseases in which antibiotic-resistant organisms played a major role, their extensiveness and effectiveness over time have not been reassuring.

In 1969, an epidemic of dysentery caused by *Shigella* swept through Guatemala infecting at least 112,000 persons and causing 12,500 deaths. The responsible organism carried an R factor that rendered it extremely difficult to treat with the traditionally used antibiotics: chloramphenicol, tetracycline, streptomycin, and sulfonamide. Since that period, the same organism has been identified in the United States where it caused two deaths among 159 cases from 1969 to 1974, most of which were along the Mexican border.

A second outbreak with a disturbingly identical antibiotic resistance pattern broke out in Central Mexico in 1972. Thousands of cases and many deaths were again reported, particularly as a result of a failure to recognize that the causative organism could not be treated with chloramphenicol. Even at the best hospitals, such as the Hospital de La Raza in Mexico City, the mortality rate was over 3 percent.

It was examples like these that led an expert in clinical microbiology to write that "We are at the point where thoughtful observers are questioning not whether we are in the post infectious disease era, but whether *on balance* society is much better off than we were forty years ago [italics mine]."[1]

The reasons for such pessimism are plain to see. While the pages of the medical journals are replete with advertisements announcing still another "breakthrough" in antibiotic treatment of infectious disease, hospital administrators are quietly admitting to their peers that they are facing unprecedented problems in infection control.

Almost fifty years after the first successful treatment with an antibiotic that was supposed to herald the end of infectious diseases as a major health problem, 3 million people in the United States, and over 150 million people around the world, are still being admitted to hospitals with infections that defy conventional treatment. Some infectious diseases, like typhoid fever, cholera, malaria, pertussis, and sexually transmitted diseases, are actually increasing in prevalence in Great Britain. In the United States, over 90 percent of these infections lend themselves, in theory, at least, to antibiotic treatment.

But while most patients can still be successfully treated with the first course of antibiotic administration, others require much more extensive regimens. In addition to a disturbingly high percentage of treatment failures, an *additional* two million hospitalized patients in the United States who never had infections in the first place acquire them simply by going to the hospital.

Dr. R. E. Dixon, a prominent internist, estimated in a special

[1] H. E. Simmons, "An Overview of Public Policy and Infectious Diseases," *Annals of Internal Medicine,* 89 (Part 2): 821–25, 1978.

1978 issue of the *Annals of Internal Medicine*,[2] that 10 percent of all acute hospital care beds in the United States are taken up by patients hospitalized with infections. The twenty-nine million days of acute hospital care costs the American public upwards of five billion dollars a year.

And while infectious disease, for some inexplicable reason, is not listed with the major causes of death (the Big Three: heart disease, cancer, and stroke), CDC officials admit that infectious disease actually holds an undramatic, but convincing, fourth place in the all-out race for the "major killer" distinction.[3]

With a death rate of 123 per 100,000 persons, infectious diseases in 1978 were almost four times more common causes of death than was the leading cancer killer, carcinoma of the lung. Also, a large but indeterminate proportion of cancer deaths are actually the result of secondary infections overwhelming the weakened immunological defenses of the terminal patient.

One infectious agent alone, *Pseudomonas aeruginosa,* is now recognized as being responsible for more than a hundred thousand infections in the United States each year. Despite the often heroic use of antibiotics, a disturbingly high proportion of patients infected with this organism remain hospitalized for protracted periods, and many of these cases are fatal. Other bacterial diseases have been recognized in recent years, notably those caused by bacteria in the genuses known as *Klebsiella, Enterobacter,* and *Serratia.* Infections caused by these bacteria are notoriously difficult to treat with antibiotics. A small cadre of clinicians is now publicly admitting that existing antibiotic therapy is severely limited in its effectiveness in treating such dread diseases, and has recommended a review of alternative approaches that hark back to the age when immunization was universally acknowledged as the key to control of bacterial infections.

In some communities, almost 90 percent of all illnesses requir-

2 C. M. Kunin and K. Edelman (eds.), "The impact of infections on medical care in the United States," *Annals of Internal Medicine,* 89 (Part 2): 737–866, 1978.

3 J. V. Bennett, "Human infections: Economic implications and prevention," *Annals of Internal Medicine,* 89 (Part 2): 761–63, 1978.

ing hospitalization are caused by infectious organisms. In one study reported in the *Annals of Internal Medicine,* the author found that 87 percent of all hospitalizations in the Cleveland metropolitan area were for infectious disease. Most of these were upper respiratory infections, heavily treated with antibiotics.

For some of the most serious bacterial infections, notably those of the blood (called "bacteremias" or "septicemias")[4] antibiotics have long been held out as the only truly effective means of treatment. The early statistics of the antibiotic era generally bear out this optimistic view. Between 1941 and 1947, the number of patients who survived from their bouts with bacterial blood infections rose dramatically. By 1947, the number of deaths from bacteremia had dropped precipitously through the widespread successful use of the sulfonamides, penicillin, and streptomycin.

But during the next twenty years something went wrong—seriously wrong. Patients who before might have been saved by a few hundred thousand units of penicillin injected into their blood stream now required millions of units. By 1967, the death rate from bacteremia had grown back to the rates of the preantibiotic era. At the beginning of the 1980s, the number of deaths from septicemia had reached 4.2 per 100,000 persons in the United States. In major hospitals throughout America, 30–40 percent of bacteremic patients were succumbing to their infections, while twenty years previously less than half were expected to die. In 1981, one hospital—the Veteran Affairs Hospital in Buffalo—reported a mortality rate of 75 percent.

In 1974, a special study group headed by Dr. Theodore Cooper of the National Institutes of Health estimated that organisms with the highest prevalence of antibiotic resistance (the gram-negative bacteria[5]) caused between 71,000 and 142,000 new cases of infection annually in the United States alone, including at least 18,000 deaths. Most of this mortality is due to three types of

---

[4] Bacteremia is distinguished from septicemia by the presence of living bacteria in the blood; sepsis can result from toxic bacterial products with or without bacteremia.

[5] Gram-negative bacteria are distinguished from gram-positive ones by their response to a staining process developed by Hans Christian Joachim Gram in 1884.

bacteria, *Proteus, Pseudomonas,* and *Escherichia coli,* which emerged as major causes of human morbidity and mortality only after World War II, where they accounted for the greatest proportion of infections among battle-injured or burned combatants. Six years after Cooper's study group made their estimates, the numbers have doubled.

Cooper's group conceded that the widespread use of antibiotics during this period for treating other infections, "clearly played a role" in encouraging the appearance and spread of blood-borne bacteria. While new hospital practices that increased the opportunity of infection, like the use of indwelling catheters, undoubtedly exacerbated the problem, Cooper's group could cite the dramatic rise of antibiotic-resistant bacteremia and pneumonia in the very young, old, and constitutionally impaired as signaling a more pervasive problem.

By 1976, gram-negative infections were found in over 1 percent of all hospital admissions, and penicillin-resistant pneumococci in about 2 percent of clinical isolates from pneumococcal pneumonia patients, where a decade earlier, none were to be found. In February 1981, deaths from pneumonia outnumbered those from motor vehicle accidents for the first time in recent history.

In spite of such gloomy figures, the production of antibiotics remains a growth industry. In 1943, there were 29 pounds of penicillin in existence. Just ten years later, 860,000 pounds had been produced. Between 1960 and 1970, U.S. production of all antibiotic preparations trebled—while the population increased by only 11 percent. A single four-year period from 1967 to 1971 shows just how much of this phenomenon was due to real growth in antibiotic productivity. During this period, the number of Americans increased by about 5 percent, as did the number of house calls made by physicians. But the amount of antibiotics produced jumped by an astonishing 30 percent!

What factors contributed to this remarkable growth? A reasonable supposition might be that a substantial number of diseases had been discovered during this same time that were responsive to antibiotics, or, that new antibiotics were streaming into the market, targeted against previously resistant infectious diseases. But epidemiologic data for this period simply do not support any such reasonable interpretation. No major new epidemics of infectious disease were recorded in the developed countries between 1967 and 1971. No new diseases were discovered that were responsive to antibiotic treatment. And, with the exception of the previously discovered cephalosporins (circa 1953), no breakthroughs in developing new antibiotics were made.

By the end of the 1970s antibiotics accounted for over 1.55 billion dollars a year in sales for the American pharmaceutical industry.[6] Of this total about 40 percent of production was used to treat the feed of livestock as a measure for ensuring maximal growth and weight gain. Of the remaining cost outlays, a large proportion went to the more expensive antibiotics. These antibiotics, principally those known as aminoglycosides and cephalosporins, are among the most costly per unit dose ever produced. In spite of their hoped-for universal effectiveness, fewer and fewer of the initially susceptible strains of bacteria remain responsive to even these "second" and "third" generation miracle drugs.

While some have questioned the fact that an appreciable portion of antibiotic production goes toward so-called prophylactic uses in animal husbandry, others argue that the remainder is much needed as a means to offset the inevitable increases in mortality and morbidity that accompany uncontrolled infectious disease. Antibiotic practice is evidently in keeping with this outlook, since between one fourth and one third of all of the patients who enter a hospital receive a course of antibiotic treatment during their stay. But an average of half of these treatments go to the less than 10 percent of patients who are on surgical wards. And only a very small percentage of these actually have preexisting infections.

The remainder, much like the livestock of our feed yards, are "prepped" with antibiotics as a means of reducing their risk of infection before the fact. The issue of such prophylactic treatment is among the most hotly debated topics of hospital wards and medical journal editorial pages and will be reviewed thoroughly in Chapter 8. One reason for such notoriety is that, through the 1970s, repeated audits revealed that more than half of all the an-

[6] International sales total about 15 billion dollars.

tibiotics used in hospitals or in general practice were either inappropriate, incorrectly administered, or simply unneeded.

In spite of growing evidence of such misuse, their prolific administration continues unabated. A pattern was begun in the 1950s whereby antibiotics that were "good" for treating one disease (e.g., pneumonia) were automatically thought to be good for another (e.g., colds). This practice continues in modified form. Now, inappropriate use may be found in the surgical wards and in office practice where pretesting to determine the susceptibility of a given organism to the antibiotic in question is foresworn. Instead, increasing numbers of physicians rely on deceptively named "broad-spectrum" antibiotics that supposedly cover any absence of clinical precision.

One of the most pervasive myths that sustains the faith in such antibiotics is the belief that their antibacterial forerunners were what curbed the major killers of the past. Such a view, held by lay persons and physicians alike, is a distortion of what really happened. The demise of the major infectious killers—infantile dysentery, tuberculosis, tetanus, pneumonia, and typhoid fever—is probably the result of a complex constellation of factors, including social, political, and hygienic ones, that led to improved sanitation and immunization practices.

For other diseases, like polio, smallpox, whooping cough, and measles, antibiotics played no role at all as immunization campaigns all but eliminated these previous scourges. Nonetheless, many public health observers still believe that the mainstay of the success in controlling infections was the biochemical revolution that permitted the isolation and mass production of antibiotics. In actuality, many of the dramatic reductions in incidence of treatable infectious disease were well under way before the antibiotic revolution had truly taken hold between 1946 and 1950, and could have exerted a downward influence.

The trends for death in children under the age of fifteen in industrialized countries during the period from 1860 to 1965, for instance, reveal quite a different pattern from that proposed by believers of antibiotics' primary role in reducing the burden of infectious disease. According to British epidemiologist R. R. Porter, nearly 90 percent of the total decline in the death rate during this epoch had occurred prior to the introduction of antibiotics. A parallel phenomenon was occurring at the same time in America. Acute rheumatic fever, one of the diseases whose control has been most often attributed to antibiotics, actually was in decline for thirty years before the introduction of penicillin or sulfa drugs. (Figure 1.) Antibiotics may have permitted the continuation of this downward trend or even have accelerated it for infectious diseases like pneumococcal pneumonia, but they certainly did not start the cycle of decline. Unlike immunization for smallpox, no antibiotic can be said to have proven successful in truly eradicating any infectious disease in modern times.

However, some of the diseases that appeared to be on the wane seem to be staging a comeback. Tuberculosis, malaria, and even pneumococcal pneumonia are more of a problem today than ten

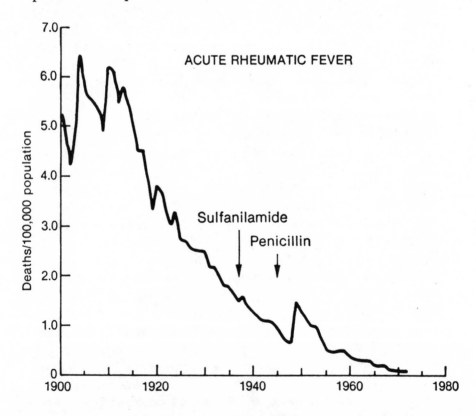

Figure 1. Acute Rheumatic Fever: Deaths per 100,000 Population—Impact of Sulfanilamide and Penicillin

years ago. Still others, like dysentery caused by *Shigella* or *Salmonella* organisms, are showing up in developing countries with new and significant degrees of resistance to a multiplicity of antibiotics. In the United States, reported *Salmonella* infections have increased dramatically over the last thirty years, and are still growing from their current levels of 52,000 per year.

To be sure, antibiotics have saved many people with life-threatening infections and promise to save still more whose existence might be compromised by premature exposure to infectious agents. Newborns, for instance, with a high risk for contracting an infection in the intensive care nursery, can be substantially protected against serious streptococcal infections by a single shot of penicillin. (The reduction of risk of infection with Group B streptococcal infections that appears to be achievable with prophylactic penicillin is not without cost since it is offset, in the first year at least, by an increased risk of infection with penicillin-resistant bacteria). In general, most patients who have serious infectious diseases caused by susceptible organisms can expect to be helped by antibiotic treatments. Their recovery times are almost always shorter than they would have been, say, twenty years ago. Except for the admitted complications of superinfections that may compromise therapy, and the hidden cost of susceptibility to antibiotic-resistant infections later, patients treated with antibacterial drugs in the early days of antibiotic use could expect to be hospitalized for shorter periods than before antibiotics were widely introduced. Or at least that is what the statistics assembled in the 1960s and early 1970s showed. Now the situation is complicated by the prevalence of cases where hospitalization is in fact *protracted* as the result of mistreatment with antibiotics or acquisition of antibiotic-resistant infections. And some dangerous infections, such as brain abscesses, are still just as fatal in the absence of surgical intervention as before—with or without antibiotic treatment!

The generally sanguine public attitude about their protection thanks to the proliferation of antibiotics has begun to pale. No one has carefully projected the true costs of relying on these agents in lieu of alternative approaches like vaccination programs. Nor is it clear that the amount of resources that have been devoted to developing, sustaining, and marketing antibiotics—

indeed creating and sustaining whole new industries—has been proportional to the benefits reaped. We are just now uncovering some of the hidden costs of making chemicals do the work of our immune systems and hygienic programs. Many old killers have been replaced by new ones. In part because of antibiotic use, diseases like gonorrhea which were once relatively trivial and curable consequences of sexual dalliance have escaped control and become major causes of sterility and serious pelvic inflammation. Organisms that used to be mere "commensals" (literally, "living at the same table") of our bodies have now emerged as entirely new threats to our well-being. Our otherwise neutral intestinal bacteria, particularly the most prevalent form, *Escherichia coli,* have undergone rapid evolutionary change under the pressure of new hospital practices and antibiotic use, and some have changed into dangerous pathogens. Casual encounters with organisms like those in the *Proteus* and *Pseudomonas* genuses were once innocuous. Today, these germs are among the major causes of death on our burn wards.

At least some of the revolution in disease-causing ability among our microscopic enemies can be directly attributed to the patterns of antibiotic use in recent years. These newly emerged antagonists are not to be treated lightly. Pseudomonads, for one, can now thrive in the very slop pails and antiseptic solutions used in the past to control them. And at least one organism has been so heavily attacked by antibiotics that it requires them to survive! Our devil-may-care attitude toward other germs with poetic-sounding names like *Serratia marcescens* led to ill-conceived programs of using them for "markers" in biological war games— possibly contributing to the increased recognition of pneumonias caused by this "non-pneumonia-producing" organism.

Unlike the questionable effect of antibiotics on the course of major infectious diseases, the dramatic impact of antimicrobial drugs on the practice of medicine is undeniable. To understand this impact it is critical to appreciate the peculiar stepwise history of the introduction of each antibacterial substance. Almost always, the general pattern of antibiotic usage in the medical profession has led from initial success and enthusiasm to partial or complete failure and disaffection. As each new agent went to work on a susceptible population of bacteria, it appeared to be plagued by the emergence of resistant forms or the appearance of unanticipated side effects. In short, almost every "miracle" drug seemed to need replacement or backup with a new one to ensure continued efficacy.

Unfortunately the complex policy implications of this pattern, so readily recognizable to experts in contemporary systems analysis, were all but lost on the first generation of pharmaceutical manufacturers. With the rare exception of the early university-based programs for developing penicillin, streptomycin, and bacitracin, or the initial contributions of researchers like E. P. Abraham and P. Newton, who developed the cephalosporin antibiotics, virtually all of the antibiotics in use today were conceived of, developed, synthesized, and eventually produced by grantees of the pharmaceutical industry, or by in-house researchers themselves. Indeed, the advent of antibiotics breathed new life into many pharmaceutical giants who created whole new operational branches within their corporate structure to generate novel—and often not-so-novel—antibiotics.

By 1974 this cyclical process of innovation and therapeutic failure led to the generation of at least three thousand different antibiotics and at least thirty thousand derivatives. Creation of new antibiotics still continues, albeit at a slower pace, with more scientists than ever devoting their energies to discovering or perfecting new chemical variants or combinations. The fact that only a handful of extraordinarily profitable antibiotics (some forty or so) are in general clinical practice at any one time suggests that factors other than medical exigency shape this marketplace.

Our seeming dependence on a constant proliferation of new antibacterial drugs belies the actually very minimal clinical requirements for antibiotics. Some countries, such as Czechoslovakia and China, effectively rely on fewer than ten to fifteen antibiotics for all of their health needs, keeping potent antibiotics like tobramycin "in reserve" for emergencies. In this country the disparity between the number of antibiotics prepared and in actual use is staggering. No more than one in every thousand synthesized antibiotic compounds has found its way into clinical practice. Even a cursory glance at Table 1 reveals the surprisingly small yield of truly effective antibiotics from their possible progenitors.

In spite of growing evidence for the relative insensitivity of contemporary strains of bacteria to the most extensively used antibiotics (e.g., penicillins and tetracyclines), a surprising number of these first-generation antibiotics remain in use today, in contrast to the characteristically short useful life (ten years or less) of other drugs. The difference, in part, rests with the ability of practitioners to escalate the therapeutic dose of most antibiotics (because of their low toxicity) to keep pace with steadily increasing nonspecific resistance.

The rather modest beginnings of the antibiotic era bely this later proliferation. Certainly, the pattern of looking for molecularly tailored antibiotics for controlling a single type of microorganism was anticipated by their discoverers. But, researchers like Florey and Chain envisioned antibiotics as being group-specific toxins. Penicillin would control "gram-positive" infections, and second-generation agents the "gram-negative" ones. The history of these discoveries suggests divergent outlooks and motives from those of contemporary researchers.

TABLE 1

Major Antibiotics in Use in the United States
circa 1975–86*

Class	Number Reported Prepared	Major Antimicrobial Chemicals in Use
Penicillins†	23,000	Amoxicillin
		Ampicillin
		Carbenicillin
		Cloxacillin
		Penicillin G
		Penicillin K
		Ticarcillin

* Source: modified and updated from D. Perlman, "Antibiotics Old and New," *Wisconsin Pharmacy Extension Bulletin,* 18: 1–4, October 1975.

† These two groups comprise the beta-lactam antibiotics.

Penicillinase-resistant penicillins		Cloxacillin Dicloxacillin Flucloxacillin Methicillin Nafcillin Oxacillin
Cephalosporins†	7,000	Cefamandole Cefatoxin Cefazolin Cefitzoxime Cefoclor Cefonicid Cefoperazone Cefotaxime Ceftazidime Cephacetrile Cephalexin Cephaloglycine Cephaloridine Cephalothin Cephapirin Cephradine Moxalactam
Rifamycins	1,500	Rifampicin
Tetracyclines	3,000	Doxycycline Methacycline Minocycline
Lincomycins	750	Clindamycin
Streptomycins	300	Dihydrostreptomycin Streptomycin‡

‡ Streptomycin is also considered an aminoglycoside.

Class	Number Reported Prepared	Major Antimicrobial Chemicals in Use
Aminoglycosides	1,000	Amikacin Gentamicin Kanamycin Netilmicin Tobramycin Vancomycin
Erythromycins	25	Erythromycin
Chloramphenicol-like products	10	Chloramphenicol
Combination drugs	unknown	Imipenem-cilastatin Sulfadoxine-pyrimethamine Ticarcillin-clavulanate Ticarcillin-tobramycin Trimethoprim-sulfamethoxazole

3

The Quest for Miracle Drugs

The history of antibiotic use usually dates from the dramatic discovery in 1928 by Sir Alexander Fleming of the progenitor of all the "wonder drugs"—penicillin. But the use of naturally produced products of fermentation to control infections, of which Fleming's famous mold is but one example, can actually be traced far back into recorded history—and probably before.

An Egyptian stele (or pillar) dated around the year 2160 B.C. shows a physician providing a cup of beer to Inde, a high priest. The beer, or a similarly flavored concoction, was believed to mask the bitter taste of medicines. In fact, it was likely that the fermenting yeasts and fungi that comprise the sediment in all grain-synthesized alcoholic products were the source of any medicinal effect. It is thus likely that the Egyptian physician's success can be traced to the antibacterial properties of his vehicle, rather than his medicine. Even the pre-Egyptian Sudanese were known to have used tetracycline-like preparations as shown in the tell-tale markings of fluorescent tetracycline deposits in their bones.

With such hindsight we can review the anthropological records of many prescientific societies. Some used poultices from moldy bread to pack wounds, and extracts of "spoiled" foods or drinks, and other products, like cheeses, known to have been produced through the action of molds or fungi to treat patients who appeared to have infectious diseases.

Often as not, such contaminated substances may have aggravated the illness. But occasionally, as may have been the case of the evidently successful Egyptian physician, we can imagine that the treatment worked. Many molds and moldlike bacteria in fact have rather remarkable bacteria-inhibiting abilities, a reality not lost on the early practitioners of crude therapeutic medical sciences across the centuries.

By the time of Fleming's dramatic discovery in 1928, over half a century of research and investigation had prepared the soil for further discoveries. In the 1870s, British researchers John Burdon Sanderson, Joseph Lister, William Roberts, and John Tyndall had already each described the antagonistic activity of a certain mold to bacterial growth. Not coincidentally, the mold in question was in the same genus as Fleming's—*Penicillium*. In 1896, a French medical student, Ernest Duchesne, demonstrated a similar bacteriostatic effect from *Penicillium* molds.

These investigations were accompanied in parallel fashion by the first true attempts to use one bacterial species to control another—the essence of "antibiosis." In 1899, German researchers Rudolf Emmerich and Otto Low successfully used the residues left behind after culturing a bacterium known as *Pseudomonas pyocyanea* to kill other bacteria. These researchers rushed to bring their new discovery to the attention of the medical community. But the first patients responded so violently to the toxic effects of the "pyocins" in their preparations that all further efforts were halted for fear of unleashing an epidemic of iatrogenesis.

Had Low and Emmerich's derivatives not proven so toxic, antibiotics could well have been a German not British discovery, and changed the course of history. For in both of the World Wars, infectious diseases such as typhus, typhoid fever, and malaria incapacitated and killed more troops than did the forces of the Allied and Axis powers combined. Between the Wars, the possibility that *Penicillium* molds might be desirable candidates as bacterial fighters had captured the minds of many researchers, considering the number of papers published on this subject during the period from 1900 to 1928 on this one genus. Certainly, by the end of the nineteenth century, the idea of isolating a chemical that would directly impede bacterial growth was widespread among medical researchers across the continent of Europe.

These precedents helped inculcate the belief that microscopic organisms held the answer to the human problem of infectious disease and prepared the soil for momentous experiments. The initial approach, championed by Lord Joseph Lister, was to use the organic chemicals generated by the burgeoning science of organic chemistry to control bacteria.

Lord Lister's solution was carbolic acid. Unfortunately it lacked the necessary specificity to attack the strains of bacteria which were most often associated with wound infection. More critically, the phenol itself was often a cause of coma and death if more than a small area of broken skin was exposed to an antiseptic solution.

Lister's belief in the chemical prophylaxis of infection was well received by Paul Ehrlich, who also supported the idea of synthesizing specific chemicals for combating bacterial infections. Although Ehrlich's work never really produced a specific antimicrobial substance, even after thousands of compounds were tested, it served as the impetus for major German chemical and pharmaceutical firms, like I. G. Farben Industries, to prepare whole batteries of synthetic chemicals. Indeed, I. G. Farben had synthesized a truly effective antibacterial drug in the sulfa family as early as 1908: as luck would have it, this chemical was one of the few that Ehrlich did not test.

Salvarsan, number 606 in Ehrlich's series, was his "magic bullet" for syphilis. Unfortunately, it proved to be too toxic for widespread use. Nonetheless, the quest for substances that Ehrlich described as "charmed bullets which strike only the objects for whose destination they have been produced" continued with unremitting vigor well into the twentieth century.

The sulfa drugs are the direct descendants of Ehrlich's ideas. The "Sulfa Era" can be said to have begun with the report delivered in 1935 by Gerhard Domagk at I. G. Farben's Institute for Experimental Pathology in Germany. Writing in 1935, Domagk described the use of the compound called *Prontosil* which he had synthesized in 1932 to treat streptococcal infections in mice. This drug, 2,4-diaminoazobenzene-4'-sulfonamide, was the first sulfonamide used widely to treat human infections.

Taking their lead from this initial study, Drs. J. Trefouel, F. Nitti, and D. Bovet of the Pasteur Institute in Paris were able to demonstrate that a derivative of Prontosil called "para-aminobenzenesulfonamide," or sulfa for short, was more effective and less toxic than its parent form.

The sulfonamide drugs became famous overnight and went into almost instant use in Japan (then an ally of Germany) for treating dysentery. In 1937, they were first used in the United States for treating urinary tract infections. An early derivative of the sulfa drugs called Gantrisin (3,4-dimethyl-5-sulfanilamidoisoxazole) is still widely prescribed for bladder infections, primarily because of its ability to concentrate in the urine. It is also more soluble than the other sulfa drugs, and reaches higher effective levels in the plasma.

In contrast to the line of descent which led to the development of chemotherapeutic agents, a less popular conceptual approach stemmed from the belief (championed by Pasteur and his notable Russian colleague, Élie Metchnikoff) that mechanisms of defense against bacteria existed in nature. According to Metchnikoff it should be possible to discover "natural" antimicrobial chemicals in the habitat of microbes themselves.

Metchnikoff and others at the Pasteur Institute also developed a parallel line of thought that sought microbial counterparts to the chemical antagonists. This work led Metchnikoff to develop cultures of bacteria, notably *Lactobacillus* species, which could be taken to offset, or displace, other more noxious microbes in the intestinal tract. Today, Metchnikoff's ideas are undergoing a resurgence of interest as holistic health practitioners prescribe yogurt and other *Lactobacillus* cultures to treat intestinal upsets and mild bacterial diseases, and more orthodox practitioners explore the use of bacterial antagonists to interfere with colonization by harmful bacteria.

Because of this intense interest in chemical disinfectants and bacteria-inhibiting chemicals, many researchers in the early 1900s were following Ehrlich's lead. By the early 1920s, the fact that some *Penicillium* molds had direct bacteria-killing properties had already been discovered by two French scientists, André Gratie and Sara Dath.

But neither of the French scientists had the prescience to test systematically the molds' bacteriostatic effects. In an unremarkably titled article that appeared in the British *Journal of Experimental Pathology* (Vol. X, No. 3, for 1929), Fleming described fully the tests that had not yet opened the eyes of his colleagues to the clinical potential of a derivative of *Penicillium*. Fleming's article "On the Antibacterial Action of Penicillium, with Special Reference to Their Use in the Isolation of *B. Influenzae*," was received for publication on May 10, 1929, and began with these modest words:

> While working with staphylococcus variants a number of culture-plates were set aside on the laboratory bench and examined from time to time. In the examinations these plates were necessarily exposed to the air and they became contaminated with various microorganisms. It was noticed that around a large colony of a contaminating mold the staphylococcus colonies became transparent and were obviously undergoing lysis.[1]

With this rather understated beginning, the medical profession was introduced to what was to become the most potent and nontoxic chemical agent yet known for controlling bacterial infections. (Laboratory scientist to the end, Fleming was more impressed at this time with the ability of his culture broths to help

[1] A. Fleming, "On the Antibacterial Action of Penicillium, with Special Reference to Their Use in the Isolation of *B. Influenzae*," *Journal of Experimental Pathology*, 10: 226–36, 1929.

in isolating otherwise rare, penicillin-resistant bacteria, than he was with its therapeutic powers!)

Fleming's discovery has been the subject of renewed interest. As Fleming himself described the events, he had the good fortune to have been culturing a batch of staphylococci that became contaminated with mold spores. These spores, arriving serendipitously through an open window in his laboratory, germinated on the agar plate containing the staphylococcus bacteria, formed the special single-cell roots called "mycelia" that produce penicillin, and thereby destroyed the surrounding bacteria.

In a marvelous piece of British detective work, Sir Ronald Hare, Emeritus Professor of Bacteriology at the University of London, pieced through the record and found this story unconvincing. For one thing, *Penicillium* intentionally seeded onto plates where staphylococcus had formed visible colonies rarely if ever succeeds in growing at all. More to the point, visitors to Fleming's laboratory reported that he *never* left the window open! So how was the famous result obtained?

Hare tried to duplicate the conditions of Fleming's laboratory. First, Hare tried inoculating an agar dish with both staphylococci and the suspected mold and placing the mixture in an incubator at 37° C (about body temperature). No effect—the staphylococci simply outstripped the *Penicillium* and grew out over the dish's surface. Hare knew that molds like *Penicillium* grow as well or better at lower temperatures where bacteria like the staph microbes hardly grow at all. Could the plate actually have been left at room temperature? Hare reviewed his notes. Fleming had reported that he had inoculated the staphylococci just before he left for vacation in the last week of July 1928. Weather records for the period show that London had experienced a heat wave through July 27, but that on July 28, the temperatures had plummeted into the 60° F range.

So, if Fleming by chance had completely forgotten to put his fateful agar plate away just before vacation, and instead had left it out on his laboratory bench top, it was possible—just possible —that the climatic change was the critical factor.

Hare found that if he incubated his mixed culture between 61 and 65° F, rather than a higher temperature, the bacteria could not grow out faster than the mold—and the tiny mycelia, or microscopic roots, of the mold would produce penicillin. The large bow window in Fleming's lab could well have been the deciding factor, Hare reasoned, if it permitted the now vacant laboratory to equilibrate with the unusually cool London summer air.

But we learn that the moldy plates were in fact discarded just before Fleming's return. How could he have had the insight to retrieve this one culture from the waste pail? This answer comes in the person of Dr. D. M. Pryce, who unexpectedly visited the laboratory just on Fleming's return and asked to see what he was up to.

Noticing the discarded plates, Fleming picked one up for inspection and discovered the now famous clear zone around the growing bacteria where they came in contact with the colony of *Penicillium*. In Fleming's own words, "When I saw the bacteria fading away, I had no suspicion that I had a clue to the most powerful therapeutic substance yet found to defeat bacterial infections in the body. But the appearance of the culture plate was such that I thought it should not be neglected."[2]

In this characteristic piece of understatement, Fleming reveals the phenomenon that every truly creative scientist knows: Discovery favors a prepared mind. No matter that the variety of mold itself was extremely rare (it was being studied in the same building by Dr. C. J. La Touche, just down a connecting stairwell); no matter that the fluke in the weather was the *only* way that the mold could have worked; no matter that Fleming's absent-mindedness was a key ingredient—the reality of serendipitous discoveries like these is that they are conditioned by a cultural readiness as well as by insightful perception.

Through Hare's detective work we know that Fleming was extraordinarily lucky. But we also know that if he had not chanced on penicillin, any one of a dozen different laboratories would have made the same discovery in a matter of a few months or years. The fact was, the world was ready for penicillin.

Recognizing the potential significance of his discovery, Fleming

[2] First Lister Lecture, Edinburgh, Scotland, November 9, 1944 (summarized in *Lancet*, 2: 677, 1944).

published his findings as a note in the British journal *Lancet* in September 1928. During the next few years, literally dozens of other scientists picked up the quest for these inhibitors of bacterial growth. Like Fleming, the first wave of researchers recognized that the soil itself might serve as an almost limitless reservoir of organisms that competed with their bacterial counterparts through a kind of miniature chemical warfare. Among the leaders during this time was René Dubos, of the Rockefeller Institute in New York. There, Dubos discovered Gramicidin in 1939, a potent but highly toxic antibiotic with dramatic effects against gram-positive bacteria. Selman Waksman of Rutgers University in New Jersey focused attention on another group of microorganisms, the actinomycetes. By the early 1940s, when penicillin was just reaching clinical application, Waksman had found or named over twenty different potential antibiotics. Ten years later, Waksman and his co-workers had identified two hundred, including streptomycin, chloramphenicol, tetracyclines, and erythromycin.

The credit for bringing the first of these antibiotics to the point where its effectiveness could be tested on human patients belongs to Sir Howard W. Florey and Ernst B. Chain at the Sir William Dunn School of Pathology at Oxford University. Beginning in 1938, these two researchers started a systematic study of antibacterial substances. They had the perseverance and insight to seize on just the right culture medium—and just the right strain of mold—to produce penicillin in clinically useful quantities.

Hundreds of different varieties of the *Penicillium* molds had to be tested and discarded, and still others produced through the "magic" of X-ray-induced mutation then recently discovered by Hermann Muller at Indiana University, before the right strain was found that could produce clinically useful amounts of this new drug. (It took until the beginning of 1940 before Florey and Chain had enough penicillin even to think of trying to treat a patient.)

As with so many novel but unknown substances that came into the medical world at this time, controlled trials were the exception rather than the rule. Instead of "blind" clinical tests to determine penicillin's efficacy, desperately ill or terminal patients—and sometimes the experimenters themselves—served as the first "volunteers" for its powers. In the case of penicillin, it was a British bobby whose plight led to the first critical test of penicillin's antibacterial ability.

In February 1940, this forty-three-year-old London policeman had cut himself shaving. Somehow, the slight wound became infected with a strain of particularly virulent and aggressive staphylococcus. Two weeks later, he developed the first ominous signs of blood poisoning: racking fever, chills, nausea, and general lethargy. By the time he reached the attention of the hospital doctors, they held out little hope of saving him. His temperature had climbed to a dangerously high 105° F. Sulfa drugs were tried to no avail. In a desperate gamble, the attending physicians turned to Drs. Florey and Chain, whose discovery had the halls of the hospital buzzing: Could this new drug save their patient?

Florey and Chain agreed to the test. They gave the physicians all the penicillin they had. In a race against the clock, the doctors injected penicillin directly into the bloodstream of the stricken policeman, every two to three hours, day in, day out. After five days on this grueling regimen, the patient seemed to be improving dramatically—his temperature was down, his chills gone. Suddenly, to their dismay, the physicians discovered that they had exhausted their supply of penicillin. Turning to Florey and Chain, they were met with total disbelief: Did not the physicians know that they had used up all the penicillin in the world?

While Florey's laboratory assistants labored to extract still more of this precious substance, the policeman began to relapse. By the time enough new penicillin was available, it proved to be too late. The London bobby succumbed to a fatal pneumonia.

Thus, the first clinical use of penicillin had a very different message than the one later broadcast to the medical community—and the world: if this new wonder drug was used inappropriately, an infection that might otherwise have been successfully treated could still claim a patient's life. With the benefit of hindsight, we may even say that with this first patient, Florey and Chain saw their very first case of antibiotic-resistant bacteria.

In fact, the limitations of penicillin had been suspected in 1940 when Chain and Abraham reported on the existence of a bacterial enzyme with the ability to inactivate it and surmised that the bacteria which manufactured the enzyme, named "penicillinase," would prove resistant. We can now surmise what may have happened during the fateful course of antibiotic treatments: The first course of treatment probably had to cope with a stupendous number of bacteria, considering the patient's advanced state. While eradication of most of the staphylococcus occurred readily, the remaining few bacteria included some with resistance to the antibiotic. When the treatment suddenly stopped, these resistant organisms grew back. Reinstituting the therapy at the same dose that appeared to work before, now was unsuccessful, and the patient succumbed to a massive infection in spite of the best efforts to save him.

In part, it was this failure to recognize the need for total eradication of the infectious agent when using an antibiotic which resulted in the emergence of antibiotic-resistant organisms all over the world. In the late 1930s, shortly after Japan had begun to experience dramatic success by using sulfa drugs to halt the epidemics of dysentery that were then sweeping the country, new forms of this particular form of diarrheal disease seemed to appear as if by magic. The organism in question, the *Shigella* bacterium, was soon found all over Japan and showed remarkable resistance to the previously dramatic killing power of these same sulfa drugs. By the 1950s the sulfa drugs had lost their effectiveness almost completely against the *Shigella* organism and the story of bacterial resistance to antibiotics began with a vengeance.

By the end of the first decade of antibiotic use (1941–50), optimism prevailed in spite of evidence for antimicrobial resistance to the major antibiotics then in use. Sir Howard Florey himself firmly believed that the few remaining problems of bacterial control were simply a matter of time. As to the problem of antibiotic resistance, he declared in an essay written for the 52nd Robert Boyle Lecture on June 1, 1950, that the absence of any cross-reacting resistance produced by one antibiotic for another ensured that the problem could be solved. Unfortunately, neither Florey nor his colleagues at the time could foresee the emergence of means to transfer resistance or the simultaneous selection of resistance to many antibiotics through the selection of resistance to one.

At the time Florey gave his famous lecture, the major antibiotics then in use (penicillin, streptomycin, Chloromycetin or chloramphenicol, Aureomycin, and Terramycin) were considered sufficient to control the majority of infectious diseases, and problems in their therapeutic use centered more on their toxicity than in the resistance of bacteria to their killing or inhibiting actions.

A resurgence of enthusiasm for antibiotics came with Selman Waksman's inspired guess that certain other soil microorganisms might have evolved the evolutionary knack of countering their microscopic foes with chemicals. In the wake of sulfa's failures, Waksman's contemporaries successfully isolated a host of antibacterial drugs from just one protean soil species, the *Streptomyces*. Streptomycin, the progenitor of antibiotics produced from soil organisms, was effective in treating early cases of tuberculosis.

In 1947, a *Chloromycetes* organism was isolated near Caracas, Venezuela, that proved to be the source of chloramphenicol, one of the most potent antibiotics known. But like sulfa-treated organisms, infectious disease bacteria treated with streptomycin and later chloramphenicol rapidly acquired resistance.

One of Waksman's contemporaries, the Italian researcher Giuseppe Brotzu, had a similarly inspired hunch that again appeared to save the day. He reasoned that so many potentially harmful microorganisms were being dumped into the Mediterranean in raw sewage, that native marine microorganisms might have developed antibiotics as a means of self-defense, as did Waksman's *Streptomyces*. Scouring the waters off the coast of Sardinia, Brotzu zeroed in on the town of Cagliari, whose outflow was notorious for its noxiousness.

Brotzu's intuition proved correct. In 1945 he isolated a fungus in the genus *Cephalosporium* that was later found to produce a novel chemical with antibiotic properties. This antibiotic, the first of a whole class of chemicals which became known as the "cephalosporins," was unique in one important feature: it was resistant to attack by certain bacterial enzymes called beta-lactamases that were fast undermining the effectiveness of penicillin.

The discovery of a whole new class of antibiotics that could withstand the degrading action of most bacterial penicillinases and other beta-lactam-ring-destroying enzymes once more generated the hope that a "magic bullet" had been found. This erroneous impression was, not surprisingly, fostered by those who had the most to gain from its perpetuation, the pharmaceutical companies.

In *Profile of an Antibiotic,* a specially printed, full-color book on the cephalosporins that Eli Lilly and Company of Indianapolis distributed to the American medical profession in the late 1960s, Lilly allowed its anonymous author to foster the impression that cephalosporins (specifically Lilly's cephalothin) would be completely immune from bacterial degradation. On page 35 of this unabashed self-advertisement, Lilly makes the statement that "in lab experiments, staphylococci were shown to develop resistance to Keflin [Lilly's brand name for sodium cephalothin] slowly, if at all." Unfortunately, bacteria do not obey the rules of effective advertising, and staphylococcus resistant to cephalosporins like Keflin soon emerged. By 1981, staph had appeared with enzymes that could degrade even the newer cephalosporins Cephradine, Cephalexin, and Cefaclor.

The quest to uncover antimicrobial substances thus began as a two-pronged search. One team of researchers, most of them German, believed that control could only be achieved through the chemical synthesis of ever more potent analogs of Paul Ehrlich's "magic bullet."

A second team of French and Russian researchers, stimulated by the work of Pasteur and Metchnikoff at the Pasteur Institute, took a more ecological approach, relying on the host's own powers of resistance, developing immunization techniques, and seeking substances in Nature herself as vehicles for controlling infection.

Unfortunately, this multifaceted search became a unilateral quest for chemical rather than homeostatic or immunological solutions. The French and Russian orientation toward the body's natural defenses was largely lost in the pell-mell race toward discovery and application of antibacterial chemicals. With this loss, the world was left vulnerable to the disastrous reaction of the microbial world to a purely chemical assault.

4

How Do Antibiotics Work?

To get a feel for why antibiotics like the cephalosporins appeared to offer such great promise, it is necessary to appreciate just how they were supposed to work to thwart bacterial—and not human —cells. Although some antibiotics have since been found to have more than one mode of action, they can be roughly divided into groups based on their ability to interfere with a particular portion of the metabolic machinery that a microbe needs in order to thrive, hold itself together, or make duplicate versions of itself.

By far the most important class of antibiotics, and the one of major interest here, includes those substances that interfere with that particularly microbial ability to make cell walls. The classic example of this kind of antibiotic is penicillin and its relatives.

The primary reason for the dramatic success of the penicillins in treating skin and respiratory infections can now be appreciated: The penicillin molecule prevents bacteria from making cell walls, a common requirement for the organisms which cause these infections. Without the rigid support of the cell wall, most bacteria simply break open and die, or collapse into an ineffective heap. While a few varieties of bacteria can actually survive without these through the construction of outer membranes instead of cell walls, they rarely can reproduce to create further harm. Cephalosporins also prevent bacteria from making cell walls, but interfere with a different part of the process. The key molecular target of both antibiotics is a substance that coats the bacterial membrane known as a mucopeptide. It is units of this mucopeptide (also known as peptidoglycan) which confer rigidity to the bacterium.

Penicillins and cephalosporins appear to be able to inactivate the key bacterial enzymes, known as peptidases, which are needed to make the cross-links between peptidoglycan units, and thereby prevent the synthesis of rigid walls.

As might be predicted from their ability to interfere with the construction of cell walls, penicillins and cephalosporins are particularly effective when used against bacteria that have the most mucopeptide and hence the thickest capsules or walls. These bacteria include the organisms most often responsible for ear infections (pneumococci and *Hemophilus influenzae*), sore throats and tonsillitis (streptococci), skin infections (staphylococci), and upper respiratory infections (pneumococci, streptococci, and *Hemophilus influenzae*). Because these same bacteria pick up the commonly used Gram stain, they are termed "gram-positive" bacteria. Gram-negative bacteria are intrinsically less sensitive to beta-lactam antibiotics, in part, it is thought, because their cell walls are impermeable to these drugs.

Because no human cells make cell walls or membranes from the same materials used by bacteria, the penicillins and cephalosporins are remarkably nontoxic at the normally used therapeutic dosages. This generalization does not hold for other antibiotics whose targets are either more universal or whose mode of action pits them against some human as well as bacterial metabolic reactions.

The sulfa drugs have enjoyed an uncommonly long life as effective antibacterial agents, particularly against gram-positive infections of the urinary tract, because of their relative lack of toxicity, a fact attributed more to their rapid elimination and concentration in the urine than to their overt toxic properties. Nitrofurans and so-called "triple-sulfa" drugs in the sulfonamide class are unfortunately also among the first to lose their effectiveness because of antibiotic resistance.

Protein-inhibiting antibiotics, by comparison, are generally more toxic to the human body. Typical inhibitors of protein synthesis include chloramphenicol and one of the broadest-spectrum antibiotics used in this group, tetracycline. A broad-spectrum antibiotic can work against several different types of microorganisms; a narrow-spectrum one, like penicillin, only a few.

Chloramphenicol, in addition to being an extraordinarily potent antibiotic, is also extremely toxic for cells of the bone marrow, producing serious clinical disorders of the blood called agranulocytosis and pancytopenia. Particularly disturbing is the so-called "gray syndrome," which is characterized by weakness, listlessness, gray pallor, and hypotension in treated newborn (especially premature) infants. Though this is a relatively rare complication, chloramphenicol has led to deaths in 40 percent of the infants who were reported with this syndrome between 1959 and 1961.

About one out of every forty thousand courses of clinical treatment with chloramphenicol develops aplastic anemia. Because of chloramphenicol's toxicity, its uses are confined to treating serious diseases like typhoid fever or bacterial meningitis in children.

Tetracycline, while less toxic, avidly binds calcium, magnesium, and other essential minerals in the body. For this reason, clinicians recommend against its use in pregnancy and early childhood, where it can interfere with the availability of calcium needed for normal bone growth and produce complexes that mottle the teeth.

A closely related group of antibacterial agents that include the B and E forms of polymyxin, a widely used topical nonprescription drug, has the cytoplasmic membrane as its principal target. These agents are relatively nontoxic, but poorly absorbed.

Erythromycin is related to both of these polymyxins and is still the "drug of choice" for treating diphtheria, whooping cough, and penicillin-resistant staph infections. It is also used to treat the recently recognized major cause of serious dysentery in developed countries, *Campylobacter fetus* subspecies *jejeuni,* and patients who are allergic to penicillin but who have beta-hemolytic streptococcus or pneumococcal infections.

Antibacterials that work inside the cell to interfere with protein or membrane synthesis are generally more effective against bacteria that do not pick up the Gram stain largely because they penetrate more easily through the membranelike component of the negative-staining bacterium's thin walls. Gram-negative infections include many of those found in deep wounds or pelvic diseases where bacteria survive in conditions where little oxygen is available. "Anaerobic" bacteria are the organisms most often responsible for these infections, and include *Bacteroides fragilis* and *Clostridium botulinum*, the organism responsible for botulism.

Other infections, such as abscesses of the brain or lung, often involve more than one kind of bacterium and can have both aerobic and anaerobic bacteria. Burn infections are particularly difficult to treat with antibiotics as they are caused by resilient organisms like *Pseudomonas, Proteus,* or even our intestinal bacterium, *Escherichia coli,* that are either intrinsically resistant or have been "selected" to be resistant to antibacterial drugs. (More about this below.) The newer cephalosporin antibiotics, such as Cephalexin and Cefotaxime, hold out promise as being effective against these bacteria.

Antibiotics that interfere with the synthesis or operation of the genetic machinery of bacterial cells (DNA or RNA) are among the most recently developed antimicrobial agents. Many of these antibiotics belong to the class known as *aminoglycosides,* a group that includes streptomycin, gentamicin, tobramycin, and kanamycin. Streptomycin was the first aminoglycoside to be isolated. More recent ones have been synthesized and have all but replaced penicillin in the treatment of certain infections that have become resistant. Aminoglycosides, for instance, have been used in place of ampicillin and chloramphenicol in treating *Hemophilus* infections of the brain (meningitis).

Aminoglycosides often work by binding tightly to one part of the apparatus used by cells to make protein from the instructions contained in the DNA and RNA. One problem posed by this mode of action is that the binding site is so specially constructed that a single genetic change in the bacterium can render the aminoglycosides all but useless.

Resistance of this kind is responsible for making kanamycin virtually ineffective against most infections caused by gram-negative bacteria. Gentamicin and tobramycin, otherwise acceptable alternatives, are unfortunately more toxic than kanamycin.

A final way that antibiotics can act is to interfere with an essential part of one of the metabolic reactions used by bacteria. A key metabolite in rapidly dividing cells like bacteria is folic acid. Antibiotics that interfere with folic acid, like trimethoprim, and many of the sulfonamides are able to control bacterial growth by interfering with one or another of the steps in the metabolism of this essential nutrient.

Combining two chemicals that interfere with the same reaction but at different places is one of the rationales used to justify combined treatment with two antibiotics. In this instance, trimethoprim and sulfamethoxazole are combined to make a very-broad-spectrum and long-lasting antibiotic known by its brand names as Septra or Bactrim. Part of the appeal of this combination product is that it need only be given twice a day, instead of the four normally required of the penicillins (ampicillin or amoxicillin). In the case of a child with a middle ear infection (acute otitis media), use of Bactrim or Septra is often a matter of convenience rather than biological rationale. As two authors of a recent review of antibiotics used in pediatric practice have emphasized, it is unclear that this combination product is in fact much better than ampicillin for treating such ear infections.[1] Even seemingly resistant *Hemophilus influenzae*, which do not appear to respond to penicillin in tissue culture tests, can respond amazingly well to ampicillin in a child. More recent clinical studies nonetheless show advantages of ceftazidime, a new cephalosporin in treating acute otitis media caused by ampicillin-resistant *H. influenzae*.

Clinicians find it convenient to separate the activities of antibiotics into those that kill bacteria outright (called a "-cidal"

[1] H. Eichenwald and G. H. McCracken, Jr., "Antimicrobial therapy in infants and children," *Journal of Pediatrics*, 93: 337–77, 1978.

effect) and those that simply stop their growth (called a "-static" effect). In practice, an antibacterial drug can be bacteriocidal at a high dose and bacteriostatic at a lower one. The effective dose of a bacterial agent and its bacteriocidal possibilities are usually determined in two ways: The first is a test called an antimicrobic susceptibility test, in which a variety of antibiotic-containing disks are put into tubes or plates containing growth medium for the bacteria. In the case of agar plates, the technician then determines the effect of the agent by measuring the width of a clear zone around the disk where bacteria are killed.

Where dilutions are made in tubes, the technician looks for the absence of turbidity as a marker of the minimum effective dose. The latter test allows the lethality or bacteriocidal effect of the drug to be measured. Both of these tests were developed over forty years ago by the founder of antibiotic medicine, Sir Alexander Fleming.

The quantitative precision of these tests can be misleading as predictors of clinical efficacy for different antibiotics. Some clinicians have argued that when the identity of an offending organism can be guessed with reasonable, if not absolute certainty, susceptibility testing may not be necessary. Unfortunately, the rapidity with which strains of bacteria are currently changing their susceptibility characteristics makes such assumptions a risky business.

An example of such a problem can be found in the classic text, *The Antimicrobic Susceptibility Test: Principles and Practices,* by Arthur L. Barry, Director of the University of California Medical Center at Davis' Microbiology Laboratories. In 1976, Barry was able to say confidently that three common bacterial species, *Streptococcus pyogenes, Streptococcus pneumoniae,* and *Neisseria meningitidis,* could be treated "blind" with penicillin on the assumption that virtually all isolates are susceptible to penicillin. Only four years later, meningitis is often found to require chloramphenicol as well as penicillin to effect a cure, resistance to both chloramphenicol and penicillin among *Streptococcus pyogenes* has been reported, and *Streptococcus pneumoniae* and *Neisseria gonorrhoeae* resistant to penicillin have become a clinical fact of life.

The existence of a phenomenon known as "tolerance," whereby

a bacterium fails to break open or lyse after exposure to antibiotics, further complicates the interpretation of these tests because concentrations which appear to block growth may not necessarily kill the bacteria. The reason for tolerance appears to be the failure of the bacterium to produce an enzyme within the cell itself that normally destroys or "autolyzes" the bacterium after an antibiotic has blocked cell wall synthesis.

Other factors are critical in the overall calculation of whether or not microorganisms will respond to therapy, with the ultimate objective being patient recovery. Chief among these are (1) the degree of susceptibility of the invading bacteria, (2) the effective amount of the drug at the site of infection, (3) the location of the infection and its severity, (4) the condition of the patient, and (5) the use of support measures, such as surgery, to drain abscesses. While most of these issues are chiefly of clinical importance, two of them concern us here: the initial susceptibility of the bacterium and its interaction with the host.

As we shall see, all but the most innocuous localized infections initially pit microorganisms against the host's natural defenses. Antibiotics usually work by keeping invading microorganisms at bay long enough to allow the host to remove and destroy them.

If for any reason the treatment is less than effective and the infection is protracted, or if large numbers of bacteria are present and the host's resistance is impaired, rapid adaptations in the bacteria may occur (to be discussed in Chapter 6) and a second battle may have to be joined against a much more recalcitrant invader. Worse still, ineffective treatment can create a minor ecological crisis whereby the instructions for resistance are spread to kindred and even entirely different bacteria. In this way, the inappropriate use of an antibiotic is as much an issue of public health as it is personal health.

5

What Happens When I Take an Antibiotic?

To appreciate the impact of even a minute amount of a potent antibiotic on your body, you must first know something about the microorganisms that live on your body and how they got there. Although there is "only one of you," as the saying goes, "there are a lot of them."

Consider the fact that you have between a hundred thousand and a million bacteria on each *square centimeter* of your skin, a surface measured in several square meters. Where your skin is dry and exposed, as on the forearm, the bacterial population density may fall to only a thousand bacteria or less for every square centimeter. But where the skin can stay moist for protracted periods, the number of bacteria can jump by a factor of ten or more! The webs of the toes come closest to a natural habitat for human bacteria, supporting a diverse population of tens of millions of bacteria of diverse kinds. Taken all together, you are likely to carry something like a *trillion* (1 followed by fourteen zeroes) bacteria on your skin alone. (Figure 2.)

Your alimentary canal, from the stomach to the rectum, contains from ten to a hundred million bacteria for every gram of tissue. In slightly scatological terms, this equates to about a hundred billion bacteria with each defecation. Another ten billion exist from day to day in the cavities and interstices of the teeth, mouth, and gums. The final census of living microorganisms comes to a staggering one hundred trillion, give or take ten trillion, or maybe a solid pound or so of living organisms.

Now, before you rush off to the shower, let me assure you that virtually all of these uninvited guests exist in a kind of perpetual truce with the rest of our living cells. Some are distinctly beneficial. Habitual vegans whose diet lacks sufficient vitamin B_{12} soon come to carry vitamin-B_{12}-producing bacteria in their gut. Other bacteria produce vitamin K, biotin, riboflavin, pantothenate, and pyridoxine. In fact, so much vitamin K is produced in rats exposed to constant attack by the anticoagulant rodenticide warfarin, that the vitamin's clot-enhancing properties can negate the usefulness of anticoagulant killers almost entirely. (Ever ingenious, the pest control people have invented a rat poison that includes an antibiotic to wipe out the vitamin-K-producing bacteria!)

Slightly more relevant studies have shown that antibiotics can indeed knock out or depress populations of bacteria that produce valuable human vitamins like B_{12}. Indian refugees in Great Britain, for instance, have developed vitamin B_{12} deficiencies after antibiotic treatments that apparently destroyed their symbiotic relationship with one or more intestinal microflora. While it is premature to say that we have the same needs for bacteria to assist in digesting and metabolizing protein as do rats, the very fact that this possibility has been neglected in the study of antibiotic use should give us pause.

From a strictly medical point of view, however, there is overwhelming evidence of the protective value of bacterial species that naturally inhabit the body. Several major species on the skin

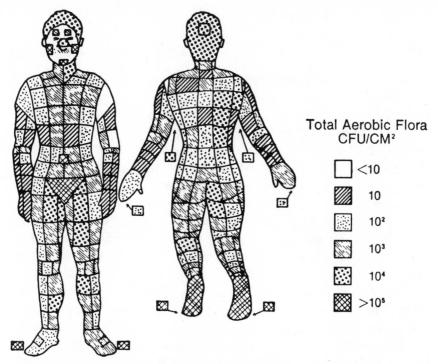

Total Aerobic Flora
CFU/CM²

☐	<10
▨	10
▦	10²
▨	10³
▨	10⁴
▨	>10⁵

Figure 2. Distribution of Bacteria on the Surface of the Skin

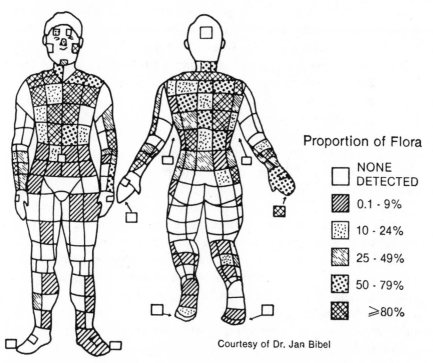

Proportion of Flora

☐	NONE DETECTED
▨	0.1 - 9%
▦	10 - 24%
▨	25 - 49%
▨	50 - 79%
▨	≥80%

Courtesy of Dr. Jan Bibel

Figure 2A. Distribution of *Staphylococcus epidermidis* on the Skin of a Human Volunteer

and in the oral cavity particularly *viridans* species of *Streptococcus,* have been shown to protect the host against harmful bacteria like *Streptococcus pyogenes,* the cause of pyoderma, impetigo, and "strep" throat, and *Staphylococcus aureus,* the major cause of skin infections. Other bacteria appear to stimulate the immune system as a kind of low-level "tonic," providing just enough new antigenic material to keep the production of "natural" antibodies humming.

Antibiotics directed against a true pathogen or disease-causing bacterium show no quarter against friend or foe alike. To the extent that we are populated with genuinely beneficial bacteria, the wholesale assault of an antibiotic can be tremendously disruptive to the normal balance of microbes on our bodies and can overcome our natural resistance to being colonized with foreign bacteria. But to fully appreciate the magnitude of this impact, you have to first gain an appreciation of the carefully choreographed process by which we are seeded with microorganisms.

Where then do all these microbes come from? For one thing, we enter the world as microbiological deserts, devoid of virtually all bacteria and viruses. The typical newborn starts the passage down the birth canal totally germ-free except in those rare instances where the mother has contracted an infection that crosses the placenta. But as the baby passes through the vagina, it picks up a number of indigenous bacteria that include staphylococci, corynebacteria, streptococci, and coliforms. We are thus rapidly colonized by a bewildering mix of new organisms. Fortunately, few of them are suited to life on the skin, and the vernix caseosa that covers the newborn protects it against serious infection from all but the most pathogenic organisms.

Nevertheless, this onslaught is not without its risks, particularly if the natural colonization process is interrupted by medical personnel who unwisely take a newborn infant away from the mother before it has had a chance to make its first efforts at breast feeding. Even if the mother does not intend to nurse, this initial contact is crucial to seed the infant with the mother's skin bacteria (rather, for instance, than those of a staph-carrying nurse). In nature's wisdom, the bonding process so essential to the psychosocial well-being of the infant appears to provide the stimulus for the immediate skin contact so necessary for healthy colonization as well.

This process of colonization, when followed carefully, proves remarkably orderly and predictable. Among the very first immigrants is the bacillus called *bifidus,* named for its resemblance to a forked stick. While an infant nurses, it ingests extraordinarily large numbers of this bacterium, which in turn proliferate in its intestinal tract. In time, it comes to make up 99 percent of the bacterial population found in the infant's feces. After the first year, its levels fall, only to increase again into adulthood, when it becomes but one of over three hundred kinds of bacteria in the gut. But while it predominates, it helps the newborn to stay relatively free of harmful pathogens by making the intestinal contents acidic and, in as yet unknown ways, suppressing the growth of harmful bacteria. Late arrivals include staphylococci, club-shaped bacteria called "coryneform" bacteria or diphtheroids (for their resemblance to the diphtheria-causing bacteria), and various bacilli.

Others continue to populate the skin through puberty and adolescence. With the hormonal storms that accompany these changes come major frame shifts in the types of bacteria that predominate, especially on our skin. Special bacteria known among scientists for their ability to release propionic acid—and to the public for their association with acne—increase in massive numbers in the sebaceous or fat glands that surround each hair follicle in the skin. These bacteria are in fact distinctly beneficial, protecting the skin and mucous membranes of the mouth and throat from genuinely harmful bacteria like *Streptococcus pyogenes* and *Staphylococcus aureus.*

One of the principal denizens of our skin, the *Micrococcus luteus* bacterium, affords clinically significant protection against several of these more dangerous bacteria. Another bacterial ally, *Streptococcus mutans,* appears to offset its more harmful relative, the *pyogenes* variety. And at least 20 percent of us carry members of the *Bacillus* family, natural producers of antibiotics called the bacitracins. (Next time you pick up a tube of antibiotic cream, check the ingredients—you will probably find bacitracin as a major component.)

The speed with which this original colonization occurs is bewildering. Within the first day of life the skin is already covered with a thin film of bacteria. In looking just at the skin of the arm pit, six thousand bacteria can be found on every square centimeter in day-old newborns; this number rises to twenty-four thousand by five days and reaches a plateau of eighty-one thousand by the ninth day of life.

When this extraordinary process is impeded or the chain between infant and mother broken, the results can be catastrophic.

One study showed that a single nurse who carried a dangerous strain of staph in her nose contaminated nine out of thirty-seven babies that she handled within twenty-four hours after birth. A second group of thirty-one babies that had already been colonized by a more benign strain emerged from their contact unscathed. They had already been colonized and hence were resistant to invasion and resultant staph infection.

Newborns placed in the semisterile environs of a neonatal care unit provide a natural experiment to test the hypothesis that separating the baby from its mother results in different—and more dangerous—patterns of colonization.

One such test was done in 1970 by a group of physicians at the Children's Hospital Medical Center in Boston, Massachusetts. The pediatricians at the hospital were extremely concerned about the high rate of colonization of neonatal intensive care unit (NICU) babies with disease-causing bacteria like *Klebsiella* and *Enterobacter*. Normally only 2 percent of the infants admitted to the care unit were contaminated with these species. But after two weeks 60 percent became colonized—and a month after admission, the proportion had reached over 90 percent. Their ultimate finding was that prior colonization with *E. coli* provided initial protection against such invasion—and the shorter the stay in the NICU, the better.

Similar results were seen in studies done in Leeds, England. Here a group of researchers were interested in finding out the difference between bottle- and breast-fed infants born in two different environments, the home and hospital. Bottle feeding resulted in dramatic increases in the numbers of potentially dangerous gram-negative bacteria such as *Bacteroides, Proteus,* and

Pseudomonas growing in the infant's intestinal tract when compared to breast-fed infants born in either environment. Antibiotic-resistant *E. coli* also made an ominous presence. Of the one hundred babies studied 61 percent became colonized with antibiotic-resistant organisms, a phenomenon most prevalent among home-born, bottle-fed infants.

The unavoidable conclusion of these studies is that we are biologically prepared to accept the natural bacterial colonizers that ultimately find us all; that forestalling their arrival is decidedly unhealthy; and, most important of all, their presence helps offset infections with genuine disease-causing microbes.

Indeed, the normal bacteria of the skin can inhibit an astonishing range of dangerous bacteria. The list of inhibited bacteria includes members of genuses as diverse as *Bacillus, Staphylococcus, Streptococcus, Pneumococcus, Neisseria, Clostridium,* and, *Corynebacterium.*

Armed with this survey of data, we are better prepared to anticipate the consequences of using antibiotics. Remember, that with rare exception all of the antibiotics currently prescribed are given by injection or orally, and thereby provide a systemic exposure to their effects. While some antibiotics like the sulfa drugs are poorly absorbed and concentrate in the urine, others, like penicillins and tetracycline, reach other tissues in the body normally inhabited by the microflora just described.

Just what does happen then after you are treated with a "therapeutic" regimen of an antibiotic? Let us take a common occurrence: your child complains of an earache. She has a fever of 101–102° F. The pediatrician finds a red, bulging tympanic membrane: diagnosis—acute otitis media.[1] The routine prescription given by most physicians in this instance is amoxicillin, a drug closely related to ampicillin, in the penicillin family. Many pediatricians will speak from long experience with this widely accepted treatment for a common infection in children. They promise swift

[1] Unfortunately, it is not uncommon to find pediatricians who are willing to make this diagnosis over the phone, with the accompanying risks of unnecessary antibiotic treatment for a more benign infection (e.g., otitis externa), or worse, the failure to diagnose a still more serious one.

improvement if the child simply follows the ten-day regimen of four treatments divided equally over each twenty-four-hour period. (As a father who has tried to follow such a regimen, I can commiserate with parents who have tried to give four doses of *any* drug every six hours!) Most infants so treated improve after forty-eight to seventy-two hours of antimicrobial therapy, but some remain ill and may require a second regimen of antibiotics, usually trimethoprim-sulfamethoxazole. (In developing countries, physicians or paramedics may not get this second chance, as debilitated infants with antibiotic-resistant ear infections readily succumb to meningitis.)

What you are less likely to hear from your doctor is that your child may experience diarrhea, or in rare instances the signs of allergic reactions to penicillin-type drugs that include rash and fever. Nor will you likely have been told that some children have developed hemolytic anemia from protracted treatments, bleeding episodes because of decreased platelet aggregation, kidney, liver, central nervous system, or bone marrow toxicity. (While these latter adverse reactions are extremely rare for penicillins, related problems are all too common for chloramphenicol.)

But even your pediatrician would be unlikely to be able to tell you about the most dramatic and consistent side effects of this drug: its devastating effect on the normal flora in and on your child's body. (I would be remiss not to add that few of these effects are likely to produce clinically evident illness; such overgrowth is, nonetheless, potentially critical in children with impaired immunologic systems, and pose risks of antibiotic-resistant infections for all children should a second course of penicillin be needed for a later illness.)

The most immediate impact of the very first doses of amoxicillin are felt in the intestine. There, many types of bacteria are drastically reduced in numbers. Some, like the *Clostridium* and *Streptococcus* varieties, rebound almost immediately—but with a difference. They are, at least for the short run, almost always resistant to the drug that is being used. More beneficial bacteria, like the milk-fermenting lactobacillus types, are almost always completely destroyed. More resistant but less desirable bacteria (including some with disease-causing abilities elsewhere in the body), begin to proliferate as more "living room" is created by the death of their normal competitors.

Among the new opportunists is a bad actor known as *Candida albicans,* a yeast that can cause serious infection of the vagina should that area become contaminated. Another is *Clostridium difficile,* a pathogen that can cause a fatal inflammation of the lining of the intestine known as pseudomembranous colitis. In the mouth, benign and otherwise protective varieties of *Streptococcus* bacteria begin to die off, increasing the risk of an overgrowth by strep varieties more likely to cause disease. The likelihood of such overgrowth increases if a second round of antibiotics is given.

Fortunately, very little of the penicillin that you take by mouth actually gets to the skin, and its flora remains virtually unchanged. But if we now move on to a second example, you will see that the skin is not always spared.

On one occasion, I found myself with inflamed sweat glands, a condition that was diagnosed as an "adenitis." Normally, such infections, like most infections of subcutaneous tissues, are caused by *Staphylococcus aureus,* or Group A (hemolytic) streptococcus. As such, they are properly treated with penicillinase-resistant penicillins. I was treated with tetracycline.

Now a large number of skin bacteria are made up of the *Propionibacterium acnes,* a normally neutral and benign skin inhabitant that has been associated (probably erroneously) with acne in teenagers. This bacterium is particularly hard hit by tetracycline, a drug championed by those who see acne as a problem calling for an antibiotic solution. (More about this below.) Unfortunately, as these benign compatriots wane, their place is rapidly filled by staph microbes that quickly develop resistance to the tetracycline. Still other bacteria, notably *Micrococcus luteus,* which holds the first line of defense in the skin against *Staphylococcus aureus,* die off and leave the field open for a potential overgrowth of antibiotic-resistant staph.

This may have been what happened to me, for much to the chagrin of my physician, and pain to me, I developed furuncles (boils) on my back during the course of my tetracycline treatment.

The initial rationale for using tetracycline for treating acne, namely, its relatively specific ability to affect *Propionibacterium acnes,* leaves in question the secondary targets of this broad-spectrum antibiotic. When tetracyclines were first introduced, intestinal bacteria were widely affected, with a dramatic change in bowel flora occurring in most people who were treated. No one appeared to notice or care when this phenomenon ceased—it was a clear indication of the widespread distribution of the genes for tetracycline resistance.

Other antibiotics now alter the intestinal flora with regularity. Lincomycin eliminates virtually all of the bacteria that require oxygen, while neomycin and kanamycin decrease the number of oxygen-requiring germs and the gram-positive anaerobic ones, leading to an overgrowth of *Candida albicans* and *Staphylococcus aureus.* Polymyxin can reduce the native *E. coli* to the point of extinction, leaving the terrain open for staph and strep organisms. Erythromycin has a similar favorable effect on streptococci, while bacitracin and novobiocin lower both strep and clostridia. Ampicillin and clindamycin, by contrast, appear to favor the growth of *Clostridium difficile.*

When cephalosporins are used for therapy, there is a similarly dramatic shift in microflora, particularly in the vagina. Here, the devastation of the natural residents leads to the overgrowth of *E. coli* and *Pseudomonas* as well as the disease-causing *Bacteroides.* Fortunately, when the antibiotic treatment is stopped, a reasonably rapid return of the natural flora ensues.

Examples like these suggest, but do not prove, that the pervasive use of antibiotics by our society is causing subtle and often imperceptible changes in the microflora with which we have evolved. With the rare exception of the gross imbalance that routinely leads to bacterial overgrowth (most common, perhaps, for yeast infections of the vagina), little can be said of the long-term consequences of this unintended effect.

That each individual's bacterial flora are part of an almost continuous whole, suggests that these effects cannot be ignored. Each time my body's staph are confronted with tetracycline and develop resistance, the possibility arises that I may transfer resistant bacteria to less physically resilient hosts in my family—like my children—with truly dire consequences.

The very real possibility of indirect havoc of this sort is only recently being appreciated as knowledge of the insidious nature of the spread of resistance has become better understood.

6

The Whys and Wherefores of Resistance

The most revolutionary and well-known idea of modern day biology is that all living systems owe their existence to the processes of natural selection. It is less well known that this evolutionary maxim runs as the common thread through contemporary approaches to therapy in many fields of medicine. Most notably, leukemia chemotherapy has made dramatic strides in the last ten years simply by incorporating the philosophy that tumor cells have genetic variability that makes the appearance of resistance almost inevitable—unless the clinician factors resistance into the therapeutic approach. The relevance to antibiotic resistance among bacteria is self-evident, yet few infectious disease specialists who must face analogous resistance among bacteria have incorporated this fact into their therapeutic strategies.

Instead, antibiotics are used almost without regard for the evolutionary reaction of their target species. Such blindness is all the more incomprehensible considering that an evolutionary perspective forms the capstone to a hundred fifty years of epidemiologic progress in understanding the origin and spread of infectious disease.

Antibiotics, by definition, work by inhibiting or killing *susceptible* microorganisms. We now know that among the billions of germs that make up the population of any given infection, one or more individual organisms somehow "know" how to withstand a low-level antibiotic assault, survive, and if the level of antibiotic remains low or drops, go on to replicate and form a new "antibiotic-resistant" infection. Knowing how these resistant organisms come to be at the right place at the right time is one of the keys to successful antibiotic therapy. Unfortunately, the first explanations for this phenomenon were much too optimistic—and grossly underestimated the evolutionary potential of microorganisms.

It was not uncommon to hear scientists of the 1940s and 1950s speak about antibiotics "inducing" resistance. This perspective was fostered by the observation that resistance seemed to appear only *after* an antibiotic was used on a given patient—or more generally in the population as a whole—for some protracted period. This "induction" hypothesis was dangerous because it engendered the false hope of discovering a means to prevent antibiotic resistance through the development of "non-resistance-inducing drugs." It also allowed the true genetic basis for resistance to go unrecognized for many years, and with it, the perpetuation of ignorance of the actual mechanism by which bacteria spread resistance information beyond the boundary of a single organism.

At the core of the misconceptions of those who favored the induction hypothesis was the conviction that bacteria could become resistant only by being exposed to less-than-effective levels of antibiotic. Such persons refused to entertain seriously the possibility that bacteria could exist with the information needed to resist an antibiotic's effects *before* antibiotics were in use.

Through the unwitting foresight of a handful of scientists, the materials to test this hypothesis were there for the asking. Several major bacteriological laboratories in the 1940s and 1950s routinely preserved their specimens through a process that kept the bacteria in a state of "suspended animation." Through careful freezing and drying, cultures of *Escherichia coli* were on hand that dated back to the early and mid-1940s—before antibiotics were in widespread use, and before the patients who donated the bacteria had themselves been exposed to the antibiotics in question. In 1967, a 1946 vintage *E. coli* was reconstituted and put to the test: would it or would it not prove to have resistance genes?

Of course, a negative result would not disprove the possibility that resistance could precede the application of antibiotics. But a positive test would almost clinch it. To the grateful astonishment of the perspicacious young scientist who tested this idea, the culture proved to contain organisms which demonstrated not only the presence of chromosomal genes for resistance, but also an R factor to tetracycline, a drug which only came into widespread use well after 1946!

Similar explorations for antibiotic-resistant genes took other researchers to the far corners of the globe where populations existed that had never been treated with antibiotics. If antibiotic-resistance genes only appeared as an aftermath of antibiotic exposure, then the naturally occurring organisms of these far-flung groups of people would almost certainly be free of resistance genes. On the other hand, if such genes were natural parts of the genetic makeup of microbial communities, then it should prove possible, albeit difficult, to find those genes even among peoples who had never received antibiotics—or had never been in contact with others who had.

A group of anthropologists and physicians had a rare opportunity to test this proposition on a trip to Malaita Island, a small, sparsely inhabited atoll in the Solomon Island group in the South Pacific. After obtaining stool samples from a cross section of the population they were able to culture the bacteria back in the United States. To their surprise the Malaita Islanders, who had never been exposed to antibiotics—or to people who themselves had been exposed to antibiotics—had R factors to both streptomycin and tetracycline among their intestinal bacteria! Findings like these offer one explanation for the rapid appearance of resistance to cholera in the tropics: It may well be that the native populations, like the Malaitese, already bear R factors!

More critically, for final corroboration of the hypothesis of preexistent resistant genes, the isolated R factors work the same way in inhibiting the bacteriocidal activity of antibiotics as do the R factors, which regulate the expression of classic, postuse antibiotic resistance.

These epidemiological observations suggested, but did not quite prove, an important point about the origin of resistance genes, namely, that the antibiotic itself serves merely to create the conditions which favor the outgrowth of preexisting antibiotic-resistant organisms, and does not induce others to acquire the resistance state.

However, the only way to prove the existence of any antibiotic-resistant organisms is to expose the virgin organisms to a drug and then demonstrate their presence among their nonresistant congeners. A classic "Catch 22"! Since we seem to need to use antibiotics in order to demonstrate the existence of organisms with antibiotic resistance, we encounter the uncertainty principle that says you cannot observe some phenomena without changing them.

In the case of the Solomon Islanders could it not be just as true that it was at the very time of testing with a fresh batch of tetracycline that the antibiotic-resistant forms were induced? As long as it was necessary to expose test plates to the antibiotic in question in order to detect resistant organisms, it was impossible under ordinary laboratory conditions to rule out the possibility that the antibiotic itself induced resistance.

To exclude this possibility, an ingenious set of experiments was designed by Nobel Laureate Joshua Lederberg. An apocryphal story is told of the origins of his insight. After Lederberg struggled with the seemingly impossible problem of testing the hypothesis of the origins of antibiotic-resistant genes, he found himself lost in thought one night while at a dance with his wife. The problem was apparently straightforward: how to tell that an organism is resistant to an antibiotic without exposing it to an antibiotic to prove it.

Lederberg had a flash of intuition, purportedly right in the middle of the dance floor. Without a word of warning to his wife he reached down and took a piece of her velvet dress in his hands, scrutinized it, and then rushed her off the dance floor. He asked her to give him a piece of the hem, cut a circle of velvet exactly the size of the Petri dish which he had growing with a pure culture of bacteria, and rushed to his laboratory. There he lifted the lid of the culture dish and tamped the velvet circle down gently on the surface. Having dipped each velvet fiber into the solid agar surface, he now had a thousand or so microneedles, each tipped with bacteria from one part of the dish. He immediately took the velvet and transferred the bacteria to an uninoculated dish, filled with the same agar as in the first dish.

In this way he used the hairs of the velvet as we would use miniature paintbrushes. Each one which touched the surface of the dish picked up a few bacteria, and, in placing the circle onto the new, clean plate, Lederberg was able to transfer a sample of virtually every colony of bacteria which grew on the first plate. In this way Lederberg created a "replica plate" of his original colony which faithfully reconstructed the geographic distribution of all of the various bacteria.

All that remained was to expose either plate to an antibiotic such as streptomycin and to mark on a circular transparency the exact location of the surviving colonies of bacteria.

By keeping the exact orientation of the transparency and moving it to the unexposed plate, Lederberg was able to make a prediction: either he would be able to anticipate precisely where he could find the antibiotic-resistant bacteria, or he would miss, except for random overlaps of colonies.

The first prediction would bear out if the genes for antibiotic resistance preexisted in the bacterial population. The second would occur if they did not. If the drug itself induced resistance, Lederberg reasoned, the location of the bacterial colonies that would survive his antibiotic test would be random and therefore different on both plates; if the resistant bacteria were already there, the surviving colonies on the replica plate should look identical to those on the original.

After repeating the experiment many, many times, Lederberg

was satisfied with the direction of the results: It was almost always possible to predict where most of the resistant bacteria would appear on the replica cultures. Bacteria that appeared anew on the replica plates could be explained by the spontaneous occurrence of novel mutations to antibiotic resistance.

In this way Lederberg was able to prove, as early as 1952,[1] that bacteria in fact already "knew" how to be resistant to antibiotics before antibiotics were ever used by human beings. But this conclusion raises almost as many questions as it seems to answer.

Why should bacteria have had genes to render antibiotics useless before antibiotics were even invented? The answer to this perplexing question is actually quite straightforward. If you think about the origins of antibiotics you will recall that they were discovered by isolating substances which were released by molds or other fungi that grew in the same environment as bacteria.

It has since been proven that the survival of many of these molds depends on their successful competition with the bacteria with which they cohabit. Bacterial species which were to prove capable of surviving the deleterious conditions created by the molds were generally those which had acquired the special genetic factors for resistance, thus permitting their perpetuation in the face of the noxious antibiotics. By this process of natural selection, the "pressure" of the antibiotics favors those bacteria which already have the genetic machinery for survival under the conditions of the natural world.

The selection pressure of specific antibiotics may be augmented by drugs like the antihistamines which also have unplanned antibacterial effects. So pervasive are these two classes of pharmaceuticals that their combined use has undoubtedly exerted an enormous force on the evolution of bacteria. Partial support for such a hypothesis comes from the observation that the nonspecific (i.e., not enzyme-mediated) resistance of bacteria to antibiotics has gone up dramatically. Between 1946 and 1971, the lowest concentration of antibiotics needed to inhibit bacterial growth of

---

[1] These experiments were performed jointly by Joshua with his wife Esther: (J. Lederberg and E. M. Lederberg, "Replica plating and indirect selection," *Journal of Bacteriology*, 63:399–406, 1952).

S. aureus or *E. coli* has increased sixfold. This insensitivity to antibiotics appears to represent an overall group response of some bacteria to antibiotics, and should be distinguished from the highly specific resistance to antibiotics mediated by enzymes.

With hindsight, it is evident that enzyme-mediated antibiotic resistance would be a natural component of the bacterial populations that besiege and live with humans. But it was not until 1975 that this predictable truth was confirmed. It was in that year that Dr. S. Selwyn, a British microbiologist, demonstrated that the micrococcus so prevalent on the skin produces its *own* antibiotics as a means of defense against other bacteria.

What was previously unappreciated and strangely unanticipated became clear: as with soil microorganisms, the microscopic inhabitants of the human skin surface also elaborate antibiotics as a routine part of their chemical repertoire. When we get a fungal infection of the skin—athlete's foot is a prime example—we can now explain the mysterious appearance of resistance factors among our normal bacteria to penicillin: This antibiotic is produced by the mycelia (root system) of the fungi, and our "natural" bacteria have evolved resistance in order to survive.

Explanations such as these work fine for antibiotics that are derived from cultures of molds, but how do they account for the apparent anticipation by bacteria of entirely newly synthesized antibiotics for which there are no natural analogs? Certainly those who made the first semisynthetic, penicillinase-resistant antibiotics, like oxacillin and methicillin, firmly believed that they were going to solve the resistance problem with their novel products. Yet even these scientists took their leads from the structure of antibiotics found in nature. These structural similarities virtually ensured that the enzymatic or cellular protections which worked against the parent antibiotics would also work against synthesized ones.

Thus we are all exposed to antibiotics through natural processes during our lifetimes. Such exposure probably creates the natural reservoir of resistant organisms that flare up when their more susceptible compatriots are inhibited by a clinical course of antibiotic treatment. Evolutionary mechanisms explain both the origins of antibiotic resistance, and the emergence of antibiotic-resistant bacteria.

Up until now, we have been talking about the information for resistance as it is carried on the bacterium's own chromosome. But bits of this genetic material can break off and be incorporated into "satellites" of this chromosome known as plasmids. There are thus *two* kinds of antibiotic resistance: *chromosomal* and *R-factor*-mediated.[2] A similar, though more complex, evolutionary argument thus holds for the "plasmids" or R factors on which bacteria carry antibiotic-resistance genes for explaining why those genes eventually became widely disseminated in the bacterial world. If you think of the plasmids as living organisms in their own regard, it is easier to understand how they are able to move from one species of bacterium to another. The opportunities for a plasmid's survival depend on having live hosts to parasitize. A good evolutionary strategy is thus to spread genes for resistance to the substances which potentially could decimate their hosts as widely as possible.

It will be necessary to make a technical diversion here to illustrate just how badly scientists underestimated the extent of the R-factor problem. Even after their discovery by the Japanese, R factors were given short shrift by many clinicians who believed that they would never prove to be a major obstacle to the success of antibiotics.

In the early 1960s, many microbiologists were convinced that chromosomal resistance genes could only be passed from bacterium to bacterium when they actively coupled in a process known as "conjugation." During this microcosmic sexual interlude, bacteria couple with special organelles known as sex pili, and pass their genetic material through an otherwise impervious

---

[2] A key component of resistance has recently been described which augments these two major mechanisms. Based on the existence of DNA sequences which can jump from one DNA molecule to another (called "transposons"), *transposable* resistance may be the most rapid—and dangerous—form of dissemination of all, since it permits resistance genes to move readily between chromosomes and R factors and hence into the microbial world at large.

cell wall. Were this the only way that antibiotic resistance could move through the bacterial world, things would be bad enough, but the situation proved to be much worse.

R factors rely on a much more rapid and explosive technique for their dissemination. They can be carried from bacterial cells when the cells are infected with a special virus known as a bacteriophage or related viruses (called transduction), or more rarely, when they happen to be broken open or "lysed." (Figures 3 and 4.) This can happen under a very limited variety of natural circumstances, which lead to the spraying of raw genetic material into the microenvironment. The genetic material so released can

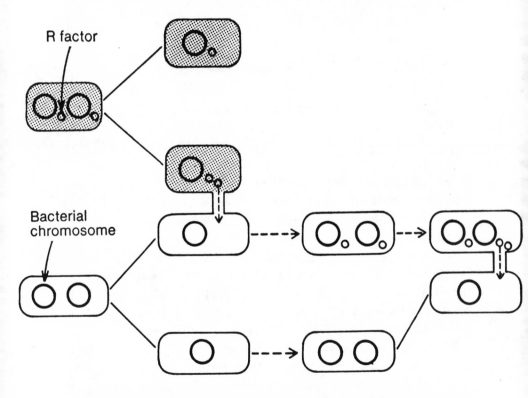

Figure 3. INFECTIOUS DRUG RESISTANCE, involves transfer of the R (resistance) factor. A cell of a resistant strain *(shaded)* comes in contact with one of a sensitive strain *(white)*; one of its R factors *(small circle)* replicates and a copy passes through a pilus to the sensitive recipient.

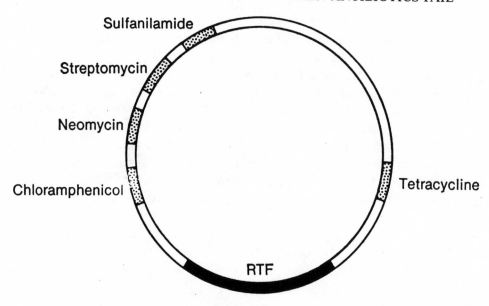

Figure 4. MAP OF *R* FACTOR shows a closed loop. There are five
determinants *(shaded)* of resistance to five different drugs. There is
also a determinant, the resistance-transfer factor *(black),* that
controls the ability of the *R* factor to replicate and be transferred.

be picked up by other bacteria. The earliest version of the process,
known as "transformation," was discovered in 1943 by Oswald
Avery and led to the conclusion that DNA was the genetic
material.

But it was at least twenty years later that the related phenomenon by which plasmid DNA can be transferred was recognized as
the major natural vehicle for special genetic transfers among the
bacteria. Now we know that transduction is the major method by
which the R factors in *Staphylococcus* are exchanged.

R factors can also duplicate themselves within the bacterium
itself, making multiple copies of their own chemical instructions
—and in the process doubling, trebling, and even multiplying by
over twentyfold the extent of the hazard to antibiotic-using
clinicians and their patients. Such duplication of R factors seems
to occur under the influence of antibiotics themselves, leading to
the gross "amplification" of the very gene sequences that are built

to destroy the antibiotic molecule. For instance, in one experiment, each single staph organism exposed to chloramphenicol and streptomycin developed on the average four to six copies of the R factor for resistance to the chloramphenicol molecule—and over twenty-two copies for breaking apart the streptomycin molecule!

A further complication of the story is the link that has recently been discovered between the genes for resistance and those for making some bacteria more virulent. Another disturbing finding is the close physical association between different resistance genes. The R factors that are enhanced by the use of chloramphenicol thus also carry another threat—they are right next to the ones that cause resistance to streptomycin, spectinomycin, and ampicillin. In practice, this means that whenever chloramphenicol is used in a way that selects for resistant bacteria with R factors, there is a good chance that the R factors will concurrently carry resistance genes to at least three other major antibiotics—and so on for each of the other antibiotics. This phenomenon creates a very serious problem in which forces that enhance the spread of resistance to one antibiotic simultaneously incorporate resistance to four others!

Add to this already complex picture the fact that R factors can replicate independently of the bacterial chromosome while inside the bacteria, and we have a scenario for disaster.

Keeping up with this immense genetic circus has proven extremely difficult, perhaps explaining in part the initial lack of concern among the medical profession, traditionally the first to sound the alarm when a drug reveals unanticipated side effects. More disturbingly, the details of the complex ecological relationships that sustain these R factors have yet to be elucidated. R factors that carry genes for resistance to human antibiotics have been found in livestock, poultry, and even cultured plants! Fish being raised in aquaculture have bacteria that harbor R factors, and so do domestic and wild birds.

Even after the true origins of resistance were known, many researchers still believed that resistant organisms posed a substantially smaller hazard to human health than did their parent strains. The theoretical argument was that the addition of the extra genetic material essential for the ability to resist antibiotics would prove incompatible with the genetic "balance" required to do us harm. The R factors that confer multiple resistance, it is argued, can only diminish the disease-causing properties of their bearer strains.

The presumption is that such extraneous genetic material "unbalances" the bacterial genome and thereby handicaps the bacterial host. Such extra genetic baggage is thought to reduce the virulence of the host, i.e., its ability to initiate, spread, and produce serious infection. Among the protagonists of this view is microbiologist Bernard Davis of the Harvard School of Medicine. Carrying the extra genetic load of an R factor does indeed reduce the vitality of some microbes—and makes them genetically less efficient than their R-factor-free compatriots—but *only* (and here is the rub) in the absence of antibiotics.

For a thirty-year period from 1945 to 1975, researchers faced with mounting evidence of the extent of antibiotic resistance in bacteria thus consoled themselves with the thought that resistance and disease-causing ability were incompatible. As late as 1975 an eminent researcher, Professor R. W. Lacey, declared in an article in *Bacteriology Reviews* that antibiotic resistance and pathogenicity simply did not coexist in any strain of staphylococci.

Obviously if bacteria could not be both disease causing and resistant to a spectrum of antibiotics at the same time, the risk that multiple resistance posed to human health could be downplayed. Unfortunately, the evidence simply was not there to support such a comforting belief.

Just when this orthodox view appeared to hold sway, new data cast a disturbing new specter across the scene.

At the St. Paul–Ramsey Hospital in Minneapolis–St. Paul, Minnesota, researchers examined over a hundred patients with staph infections to determine whether the course of their hospitalization could be related to the presence of antibiotic resistance in their bacteria. To their surprise, they discovered that the patients whose staph were antibiotic resistant had fared *worse* than those patients whose staph were presumably more dangerous because they lacked antibiotic-resistance genes.

In fact, infection with a resistant staph infection prolonged hospital stays forty-three days longer than did an infection with nonresistant staph. More alarmingly, these researchers found that patients with resistant infections had higher overall mortality rates than did those whose infections were susceptible to antibiotics.

As to the cause of this most serious situation, the researchers could only point out the obvious: a much larger portion of the patients who got the more serious resistant staph infections had previously been treated with antibiotics than had the patients whose infections were responsive to treatment (81 vs. 38 percent, respectively).

In a display of unusual candor for physicians, the St. Paul clinicians admitted that they could not stop the outbreak of resistant staph and publicly chided their colleagues for downplaying the hazards of the outbreak. In particular, the researchers singled out the irrational use of supposedly fail-safe antibiotics like penicillinase-resistant penicillins or the remarkably expensive cephalosporins, whose use only increased the likelihood of transmission of antibiotic resistance.[3]

Here again, then, resistant and pathogenic strains won out over their more benign counterparts. How could this situation have occurred in the face of such otherwise enlightened uses of medical technology? At least part of the answer lies in the almost totally unforeseen way we have shown that bacteria actually avoid antibiotic toxicity and then spread that information to other microbial hosts. But yet another source of ignorance contributes to this ongoing problem: Our failure to recognize and chart the unforeseen rapidity of acquisition and spread of antibiotic resistance around the world.

[3] K. Crossley et al., "An outbreak of infections caused by strains of *S. aureus* resistant to methicillin and aminoglycosides," *Journal of Infectious Diseases*, 139: 273–87, 1979.

7

The Development of Resistance, or Why Don't Antibiotics Work All the Time?

Most of the time, antibiotics work best when they are prescribed judiciously and with attention to the particular susceptibility of the organism being attacked. However, when antibiotics are prescribed without adequate testing to determine the vulnerabilities of the infecting organism, or when the infection has already gone on a long time, problems are the rule and not the exception. As we have seen, one of these problems is the emergence of new strains of bacteria that are resistant to the particular antibiotic being used.

The kinds of infections where this event can occur are legion. They include infections of the heart valves, bone, kidney, and deep, soft tissues of the body. Other factors that contribute to long-lasting, hard-to-treat infections include foreign bodies, an abscess, or an obstruction. These conditions also make antibiotic resistance following treatment a more likely outcome. Additionally, some bacteria, like many of those that inhabit the intestinal tract, gram-negative bacteria generally, and the ubiquitous staphylococcus, are intrinsically more likely to develop resistance than are other bacteria, like the streptococci. If it is going to happen at all, the emergence of resistant strains of bacteria occurs a week or ten days after treatment has been started.[1]

A prior course of antibiotic treatment can alter the patient's susceptibility to a second infection. When the conditions are right, such treatment can also increase the likelihood of antibiotic-resistant infections. A case in point occurred at the Texas Children's Hospital in Dallas where a group of children with serious penicillin-resistant infections caused by *Hemophilus influenzae* were found to have been twice as likely to have been treated with antibiotics in the month preceding admission than were hospitalized children who did not get this antibiotic-resistant infection.

When antibiotics fail to rescue an infected host, the causes are often multiple, ranging from poor choice or route of administration of the antibiotic to the existence of multiple infecting organisms, or simply to an inappropriate course of treatment from the start. This happens most commonly when there is a fever of undetermined origin or an unconscious patient, and the physician wants to ensure that *some* treatment regimen is indicated on the chart as soon after admission as possible, and thereby rationalizes the omission of a pretest for antibiotic susceptibility or a causative organism.

The constitution and physical state of the patient can also upset

---

[1] The rapidity and extent to which resistant bacteria can emerge during the course of antibiotic treatment is hotly contested (cf. the letters of W. V. Shaw et al., "Chloramphenicol and gram-negative bacillary meningitis in neonates," *New England Journal of Medicine,* 305: 170–71, 1981).

the success of treatment. A constellation of physiologic factors in the patient in addition to the genetic makeup of the infecting bacterium can disrupt the course of treatment. Where kidney function is impaired, not only does the patient being treated face greater risks of antibiotic toxicity, but the expected metabolism and excretion of the drug may be so badly upset as to throw off calculations of the dose needed to ensure the best treatment outcome.

But the gravest threat to patient well-being from antibiotic use is the emergence of antibiotic-resistant organisms.

In 1980, Lewis Thomas wrote, "I am worried about the future of antibiotics (as is everyone else in the field of infectious disease) if we do not continue to do research on the appalling problems of antibiotic resistance among our most common pathogens."[2] Recall that it was less than five years after introducing the first wonder drug to combat bacterial infection on a large scale, that medical researchers discovered the same chemical which previously had all but wiped out a major cause of infection had become virtually ineffective.

As was discussed in the chapter on the history of antibiotics (Chapter 3), *Shigella* was thought to be totally controlled by the sulfa drugs. By the end of World War II, *Shigella* organisms were causing rampant dysentery once again. A second wave of antibiotics was thrown against them over the next few years to supplement the sulfa drugs only to result in *Shigella* organisms with dual resistance to both sulfa and the newcomers, notably, tetracycline.

Nevertheless, through the early 1950s clinicians and public health officials remained confident that they were on top of the situation. The appearance of resistance, even double-resistant organisms, simply appeared to be chance events. Researchers surmised, and the early evidence appeared to bear them out, that resistance was the result of spontaneous mutations in the bacterium's single chromosome. These mutations, like other genetic changes, were characteristically extremely rare, occurring no

[2] Lewis Thomas, "The Right Touch," *Wilson Quarterly*, Spring 1980, p. 96.

more frequently than about once in every twenty generations—or once in every million organisms. Most importantly, as long as the genes were on the chromosome, their dispersion could be predicted.

Thus, the gene-mediated resistance of bacteria to antibiotics was believed to follow the laws of probability. If one mutation to resistance occurred for every million bacteria, then two mutational events required one million times one million bacteria, or a thousand billion organisms (1×10^{12} organisms).

Using these assumptions, researchers reasoned that with the production of the first six or seven antibiotics, the likelihood of any *one* bacterium appearing with resistance genes to all seven antibiotics was so astronomical as to exceed the total number of bacteria on earth. The one in a million chance for one mutation would have to be expanded to one in a million to the seventh power ($[1 \times 10^6]^7$), or 1×10^{42} bacteria, a number which would outweigh the total biomass of organisms on earth.

This optimistic scenario suffered its first setback in 1952. That year, a Japanese researcher, Tsutomu Watanabe, isolated an organism which was simultaneously resistant to several different antibiotics. Against the odds of 1×10^{18} to 1, a strain of *Shigella* had been found with resistance to three antibiotics: streptomycin, tetracycline, and sulfanilamide. Following this disturbing but little recognized discovery, the concept of total bacterial vulnerability to human control should have been critically reassessed. It was not. Almost imperceptibly at first, the myth of final victory over the bacterial world through antibiotics began to unravel as more and more antibiotic-resistant strains were uncovered.

The origins of concern for infectious diseases which might be slipping from medical control can be traced to the mid-1960s.

In 1964, a major international conference was held on an organism that few medical students had previously recognized from their studies as anything but a minor nuisance.[3] The conferees agreed that they were facing a major international emergency. I

[3] National Conference on Salmonellosis, March 13–14, 1964 (Proceedings published March 1965, Public Health Service Pub. No. 1262; U. S. Govt. Printing Office, Washington, D.C., 1965.).

can remember vividly the first stirrings of concern among the medical profession for this particular organism as a bona fide health problem. I was a student in the Pathology Department of the University of Washington Medical School in Seattle. In 1965, an otherwise commonplace outbreak of food poisoning had caused a stir among the local commercial fishermen. This otherwise minor epidemic focus of gastroenteritis happened to be traced to a hapless seafood entrepreneur, leading to an almost comic confusion of a delicacy and mainstay of most of Seattle's fishermen—salmon—with the offending organism itself.

The Seattle *Post Intelligencer* carried a full-page story on the issue of the fishermen and declared war on the medical establishment. The targeted microorganism: *Salmonella!* After heated discussions with the microbiology faculty, the normally self-limiting nature of the infection finally took its course and the fishermen simmered down. Their catch is still considered a delicacy, and *Salmonella* still causes food poisoning—but with a new twist.

Beginning in the 1960s (and no one knows whether we were just looking harder or if it really did begin in the 1960s), something changed among the types of *Salmonella* usually linked to relatively mild gastrointestinal upsets. The story centers on a particular variety known as *Salmonella wien* (named for Vienna, the place where it was first isolated). Before 1969, *S. wien* was rarely associated with outbreaks of human disease.

The explosion that rocked the world of *Salmonella* watchers started innocently enough—a tiny pediatric ward in Algeria. There, in the winter of 1969–70, a group of children came down, like dominoes, with infant diarrhea—all infected by *S. wien*.

Perhaps the most unexpected feature of this outbreak was the mysterious appearance of antibiotic resistance. Here was a relatively nonvirulent, noninvasive organism that appeared to spring fully armed, like some mythical warrior, to meet the challenges thrown up against it. The very first *S. wien* bacterium isolated from an Algerian child proved invasive *and* resistant to four different antibiotics. This finding was all the more disturbing because *Salmonella* diarrhea is usually uncomplicated and requires no antibiotics at all.

Within the next two years *S. wien* outbreaks were reported in

France, presumably imported there by silent carriers from clinics in Oran or Algiers. By 1977, *S. wien*, with the identical pattern of antibiotic resistance, was being reported in countries as far-flung as Yugoslavia, India, Iraq, Italy, Austria, Great Britain, and Ireland. By that year *S. wien* had risen from virtual obscurity to become the predominant pathogen responsible for gastrointestinal infections throughout Europe. Most remarkable of all, according to Dr. M. M. McConnell, the medical epidemiologist who ferreted out this story, virtually *all* of the present infectious strains of *S. wien* in Europe could be reliably traced to the single group of organisms that left Algeria a mere seven to eight years previously! By 1981, the same resistance plasmid had moved to *S. typhimurium*.

The implications of such an epidemic are staggering: Is it really possible that a single antibiotic-resistant organism could achieve such a global sweep in so short a period? Dr. McConnell's findings leave little room for alternative explanations: Virtually every strain of *S. wien* isolated in Europe during the period of his study carried the tell-tale marks of the particular mix of antibiotic resistance that characterized the first Algerian strains. Recently, other strains of *Salmonella*, specifically *S. agona*, have spread in similarly explosive fashion.

In one startling example, this case showed that a major epidemic spread of antibiotic-resistant organisms was possible, a feat once thought limited to the plague bacillus or virulent strains of influenza. Whereas the plague bacillus (*Yersinia pestis*) or the flu spread (in their pneumonic and virulent forms, respectively) through air transmission, *Salmonella* must pass through the riskier (for the bacterium) and certainly fouler medium of oral-fecal communication. Although it can survive in a dry state for protracted periods, *Salmonella* characteristically are food-borne and animal-carcass contaminants that directly infect people who ingest or handle contaminated products. (See Figure 6, p. 129.)

Since we generally do not pursue the origins of bacterial infections or outbreaks with the kind of vigor shown by Dr. McConnell, we simply cannot know if the dramatic spread of other antibiotic-resistant organisms like *Pseudomonas* has not also started from one case of an inadequately treated infection, where antibiotics were used unsuccessfully and the bacterium in question simply escaped, sorcererlike, to spread throughout a hospital—or a continent.

The exact probability of such an occurrence depends on two factors: the first, the virulence and infectivity of the organism; the second, its ability to acquire resistance to more than one antibiotic at the same time. As we have seen, this last factor was long held to be a mathematical impossibility, since resistance was thought to be a slow, sequential process.

A near-fatal blow to the precepts of the researchers who believed in the rare, stepwise acquisition of resistance came in 1959. Then, in a journal little known outside of Japan, an article appeared that detailed simultaneous occurrence of the same pattern of multiple drug resistance found in *Shigella* in another species of bacteria. The idea that the genes for resistance could be inherited was not new. But the observation that it could be transmitted *outside of the species* barrier was totally revolutionary.

Professor K. Ochai and a group of his co-workers reported that the genes for antibiotic resistance could be passed intact from *Shigella* to *Escherichia coli,* the major bacterium of the human intestinal tract. It was thus possible to imagine that before a *Shigella* dysentery-causing organism could be effectively eradicated in a host, it could pass on the "knowledge" of resistance to antibiotics to a normal resident of the human intestine and from there to *Salmonella*. More critically, since *Shigella* organisms are much more readily transferred from person to person than are *Salmonella,* the prospects for epidemic spread of multiply resistant shigellosis are greater.

Rather than a genetic roulette where bacteria could be caught without necessary resistance genes by a novel antibiotic, clinicians must now accept that *any* initial bacterial success in eluding destruction through gene-mediated resistance potentially can infect members of a whole community. A game of antibiotic escalation could now begin with a vengeance whereby organisms surviving an initial antibiotic onslaught can pass on their knowledge with dramatic swiftness to another group of organisms, and from there to wider and wider circles of bacterial hosts.

Multiple drug resistance thus poses awesome therapeutic problems. Now, instead of being able to rely on a stock formula of bacteria with predictable susceptibilities to antibiotics, clinicians have to worry if the strain in question will prove susceptible to one, two, or even five antibiotics of choice, and then, what concentration will be effective.

As Dr. Grady Fort, a pediatrician at Shasta General Hospital in California, has told me, "You used to be able to treat every 'ear' [pediatrician's term for a middle ear infection] with ampicillin. Then resistance appeared and they suggested trimethoprim. But I think I've seen my first cases of resistance to this one too. Now we'll have to use erythromycin and Gantrisin, antibiotics we should be saving for more serious infections."

Others have echoed Dr. Fort's concerns. The consequences of a spread of R factors can be appreciated by reading the words of one of the codiscoverers of infectious drug resistance, Tsutomu Watanabe:

> Until recently [1967] it was assumed that the appearance of drug resistant bacteria was the result of a predictable process: the spontaneous mutation of a bacterium to drug resistance and the selective multiplication of the resistant strain in the presence of the drug. In actuality a more ominous phenomenon is at work. It is called infectious drug resistance, and it is a process whereby the genetic determinants of resistance to a number of drugs are transferred together and at one stroke from a resistant bacterial strain to a bacterial strain of the same species or a different species that was previously drug sensitive, or susceptible to the drug's effect . . . each year it is found to confer resistance to more antibacterial agents.[4]

The remarkable thing about this quotation is that it was made at a time when such observations were rare, and the consequences of the discovery of infectious drug resistance were appreciated by only a small minority of researchers and public health officials. The full extent of antibiotic resistance only began to be appreciated in the late 1960s and 1970s. A respresentative summary of reports from around the world is shown in Table 2.

---

[4] T. Watanabe, "Infectious Drug Resistance," *Scientific American,* 217: 19–27, 1967.

Resistance of this magnitude was totally unanticipated. It caught the medical profession of the most technologically advanced countries almost totally off guard. Even under advanced hygienic conditions, intestinal diseases that appeared to be under control made their presence felt anew.

By the mid-1960s *Shigella* dysentery in Japan posed almost as much a public health problem as it had in the immediate postwar years. By the period 1965–68, 80–90 percent of the tested strains were proving to be multiply resistant. And each new antibacterial substance appeared to be met with another round of resistance genes in *Shigella*. In keeping with their own patterns of antibiotic use, *Shigella* in other countries like England and Australia soon followed suit. By 1970, 70 percent of the *Shigella* strains isolated in England, and by 1980, a like number in Australia, were showing multiple resistance to antibiotics.

TABLE 2

Representative Incidences of Antibiotic Resistance
in Various Countries

Country	Year	Species	Antibiotic Resistance Pattern
India°	circa 1981	*Salmonella typhi*	1.2% resistant to 7
Iran*	circa 1968	*Salmonella typhimurium*	100% resistant to 1 or more 27% resistant to 8 10% resistant to 9
New Zealand†	circa 1975	*Shigella*	78% resistant to 1 or more

°V.M. Rangnekar et al., "Plasmid-mediated multidrug resistance in *S. typhi*," *Lancet* ii, 364, 1981.

* K. Badalian et al., "Relation between *Salmonella typhimurium* and Drug Resistance," *Journal of Tropical Medicine and Hygiene*, 79: 28–31, 1976.

† R. A. Robinson, "Antibiotic Resistance of Shigella in New Zealand," *New Zealand Medical Journal*, 83: 81–82, 1976.

Country	Year	Species	Antibiotic Resistance Pattern
Australia‡	1976	Pseudomonas	8–9% resistant to 1 or more
Japan§	1977	Staphylococcus	93% resistant to 1 or more

‡ H. F. Dean et al., "Isolates of *Pseudomonas aeruginosa* from Australian hospitals having R plasmid determined resistance," *Medical Journal of Australia,* 2: 116–19, 1977.

§ H. Kakahara et al., "Distribution of Resistance to Metals and Antibiotics of Staphylococcal Strains in Japan," *Zentralblatt für Bakteriologie,* Original Article Series: (A) 237: 470–76, 1977.

The details of how this resistance emerged are important because they show the close relationship between poor antibiotic practice and the development of resistance. The first multiply resistant *Shigella* were able to withstand high concentrations of combinations of the sulfa and streptomycin or sulfa and tetracycline drugs then in wide use. The inescapable conclusion of epidemiologists looking back on this episode is that it must have been preceded by a sustained pattern of ineffective doses of one or both drugs in treating infected patients so that resistant organisms could survive and overcome host defenses. Triply resistant varieties (circa 1956) emerged following the introduction of chloramphenicol for much the same reason. And finally, *Shigella* appeared that showed quadruple resistance, combining four separate varieties of drug resistance in the mid-1960s.

This last pattern of resistance provides the kind of association that epidemiologists find highly suggestive: (1) The sequential pattern of drug resistance matches the sequence with which drugs were introduced to treat bacterial infections in a given country or region and (2) the final pattern of resistance provides a mirror of the complex of all the antibiotics that had ever been used in that area.

This lock-step pattern of bacterial resistance dogged the heels of drugs introduced in other countries as well, putting a fatal cramp in the assumption that antibiotic resistance was a random phenomenon. Clearly, something was shaping the drug resistance and reinforcing its appearance and proliferation. It thus became important to ascertain if the phenomenon was isolated to *Shigella,* and to determine if antibiotics were actually inducing the observed resistance.

Although *Shigella* was the first bacterium to be studied in depth, it soon became clear that it would not be alone among those showing multiple resistance. Similar phenomena were discovered throughout Europe, and later the United States, for widely divergent organisms.

By 1977, four facts had been unequivocally established: (1) the longer patients are hospitalized, the greater are their chances of acquiring an antibiotic-resistant infection, (2) infection of the human intestinal tract with a single multiply resistant strain of bacteria greatly increases the likelihood of other strains becoming multiply resistant, (3) R factors in humans are disseminated by international travelers, and (4) antibiotic therapy of *Salmonella* and *Shigella* diarrheas can actually increase the rate of spread of R factors.

Unlike the sequential and gradual emergence of organisms with multiple resistance which occurred in Japan, the staph strains in Britain appeared to acquire resistance factors in leaps and bounds. Triply resistant staph appeared as early as 1951 in hospitals where streptomycin, penicillin, and the tetracyclines had been only briefly used. This occurred even though studies performed a scant two years earlier showed that virtually all of the staph which were penicillin resistant belonged to only a few strains.

Most of the medical observers who have looked back at the British experience agree that it was the widespread use of antibiotics in open hospital wards that greatly accelerated the spread of infectious drug resistance. The previous error of using penicillin to treat virtually every respiratory illness even suspected of being bacterial was repeated with staph infections. Even those infections that would have responded to conservative treatment—such as lancing and draining boils—were systematically treated without any clear effort to establish patient need or the susceptibility of the bacteria in question.

The most far-reaching error was to ignore the impact of such actions on the infection hazard to the population at large. No antibiotics were "kept in reserve" to ensure adequate sensitivity for truly critical infections—and still fewer policies were made to rein in the unbridled use of the then effective tetracyclines.

By the time penicillin was in widespread use in the postwar years (1946–49), most of the staph strains in Britain were penicillin and streptomycin resistant. In the mid-1950s, almost every case of postoperative staph infection in Britain, as in Japan, was due to the triply resistant *S. aureus*. Even a totally new antibiotic, kanamycin, introduced in the late 1960s, lost its high effectiveness in a few short years because of resistant target organisms. By 1971, almost 20 percent of all *E. coli* being isolated in Japan and England were resistant to five or more antibiotics.

More ominously, some of the staph strains that emerged after antibiotics came into widespread use in Britain, namely, those known as type "80," appeared to have become *more* virulent than their forerunners which had lacked antibiotic resistance. Thus, by the early 1960s, dangerous staph bacteria resistant to virtually all of the second-generation antibiotics then in use were proliferating among hospitals in the United States and abroad.

This spread of novel resistance patterns among pathogenic bacteria was alarming enough in itself. What was doubly disturbing was the emergence of entirely *new* communicable pathogens in nursery and hospital wards. Three previously unrecognized classes of bacteria emerged in the 1960s as major new sources of hospital-acquired infections. As we have seen, these three organisms (*E. coli, Pseudomonas pyocyanea,* and *Proteus* species) had been previously identified as major sources of serious human infection only during the War.

Such bacteria had not been found in appreciable numbers in hospital settings prior to the end of World War II, or at least no one had ever detected them. Postoperative *Pseudomonas* and *Proteus* infections increased dramatically only in the period immediately following the introduction of broad-spectrum antibiotics, e.g., the tetracyclines. Their proven insensitivity to such antibiotics strongly suggested a role of antibacterial drugs in favoring their emergence.

Between 1952 and 1959, the first reports of hospital-acquired infection with these organisms appeared in the medical literature. By the 1970s, American clinicians were reporting antibiotic resistance in almost every isolated strain. But recognition of the full ramifications of these findings was slow in coming.

In marked contrast to alarms over this pattern of drug resistance in Europe and Japan, the United States was slow to awaken to the hazard posed by the growing emergence of multiresistant and insensitive organisms. Efforts to monitor antibiotic resistance were notably lacking in the United States until recently, while Japan, Czechoslovakia, and England all took action many years ago to minimize the occurrence of unanticipated outbreaks of antibiotic-resistant organisms.

Japan had established its central research repository on *Shigella* by 1960, and Czechoslovakia organized its Antibiotic Reference Laboratory in 1970. The United States, in contrast, only began to monitor the prevalence of antibiotic-resistant infections in hospitals with any degree of success in the 1970s, at least a decade after a workable plan had been developed for local use in New York State.

Early warnings of the need for surveillance appeared in the medical literature in the United States and went largely unheeded. As early as 1968, an editorial in the *Journal of the American Medical Association* warned that multiple antibiotic resistance, which was being reported increasingly in the medical research literature here and abroad, was being ignored here as a clinical problem with far-reaching epidemiologic implications. By 1966, reports of antibiotic-resistant organisms had been recorded from hospitals in virtually every major American city. But the concern voiced by medical researchers throughout this period fell largely on deaf ears.

Between 1964 and 1968, antibiotic resistance had already proved a major obstacle to effective therapy in major American hospitals. For instance, at the Methodist Hospital in Chicago, Illinois, resistance to streptomycin and tetracycline was reported in over one third of all pathogenic *E. coli* isolated in the wards there. Since this organism had become a major cause of intransigent urinary tract infection, this news was disturbing enough. But, then a second species of gram-negative bacteria that had been a cause of pneumonia in adults suddenly became a major problem in newborn infant care nurseries.

The organism, *Klebsiella pneumoniae,* proved resistant to streptomycin and tetracycline. In the first four years after its original discovery, it showed a progressively increasing resistance to the two most commonly used antibiotics for pneumonia, ampicillin and the new cephalosporins. Between 1964 and 1968, the number of *Klebsiella* resistant to ampicillin rose 50 percent, and *Klebsiella* resistant to cephalosporin went up by a third.

Antibiotic-resistant *Pseudomonas* infections also became a major problem at this same time. Notoriously difficult to treat, *Pseudomonas* proved highly recalcitrant to therapy, with only slightly more than one half of the strains isolated during the mid-1960s proving susceptible to streptomycin and amakacin. Over three fourths were resistant to tetracycline and chloramphenicol.

Patterns of increasing resistance to antibiotics became so commonplace during this entire period that drug companies began to pitch for "broad-spectrum" antibiotics that presumably lacked the proclivity to cause resistance. The U. S. Army even began an irrational and ill-fated program of intentionally placing R factors conferring resistance to major Russian antibiotics into pathogenic organisms as a "defensive" move in anticipation of biological warfare!

The full flavor of the insidious growth of antibiotic-resistant bacteria as a major health problem can only be appreciated by observing the evolutionary checkpoints that we have passed in our own lifetime. In 1950, few if any staphylococci were resistant to the major antibiotics then coming into widespread use. According to Dr. Maxwell Finland, who was among the first to alert the American public to the extent of the antibiotic resistance problem, by 1960, around 80 percent of the strains of staph that could be isolated from clinical specimens were showing resistance to penicillin, tetracycline, and chloramphenicol. Even higher indices (up to 14 times the U.S. levels) were found in France at the St-Joseph Hospital in Paris. Today, penicillin can only control 10 percent of the varieties of *Staphylococcus aureus* that it used to kill regularly.

With the introduction of the "second generation" of penicillins like methicillin that were protected against bacterial degrading enzymes, many researchers believed that the immediate problems of antibiotic-resistant staph that had occurred in Britain had been resolved. Unfortunately, shortly after their use in the early 1960s, the first staph strains in the United States began to show resistance to penicillinase-insensitive methicillin. By 1963, methicillin-resistant staph had become a prevalent problem in many American hospital wards. Fortunately, for unknown reasons, the wave of antibiotic-resistant staph strains receded in the 1970s. But serious outbreaks recurred in the 1980s, fueled by misuse of still another antibiotic, gentamicin.

In 1969, the resistance problem in staph was partially resolved by the introduction of gentamicin, a broad-spectrum antibiotic with proven effectiveness against infections caused by organisms like *Proteus* and *Pseudomonas.* Many clinicians believed that their problems could be overcome by using the newly developed gentamicin plus methicillin in combination to treat stubborn staph infections. Their plan proved dangerously overoptimistic. By 1976, resistance to this novel combination became apparent. In an alarming report in the British medical journal *Lancet,* a group of clinical researchers headed by Dr. D. C. Shanson reported the first serious outbreak of a gentamicin- *and* methicillin-resistant staph infection at a hospital.

The Center for Disease Control's National Nosocomial Infection Study also reported a serious episode in its October 1977 monthly report. The attention given to this outbreak highlighted its gravity. Between April and mid-August 1976, eight adults and sixteen infant patients at a Georgia hospital acquired a staph infection that proved resistant to treatment with the standard antibiotic regimen of gentamicin. In this case, the disease appeared to spread from the surgical staff to the newborns.

One adult died, but the newborns survived after being hospitalized for protracted periods. This epidemic, apparently the first of its kind, was also distinguished by having the antibiotic resistance appear on an R factor, thus providing vivid proof of the prophetic description by Watanabe some ten years earlier.

Another case highlights the importance of limiting the use of combination treatments. In December 1976, a gentamicin-resistant staph strain suddenly appeared in an intensive care nursery in a large metropolitan area in the United States. One child after another got sick, and could not be successfully treated. By April 1977, this strain accounted for 96 percent of all of the bacteria isolated from the ward. Fortunately, the strain in question was still sensitive to methicillin. Had both antibiotics been in use and dual resistance present the outcome might have been tragic.

Other researchers reported a disturbing increase in the size of the breach in the wall against antibiotic-resistant bacteria between 1975 and 1977. At the Manhattan Veterans Administration Hospital, clinicians isolated R factors carrying the genes for gentamicin resistance, and reported an alarming 60 percent mortality rate for patients with gram-negative infections caused by organisms that carried the factor. In a five-year span, between 1970 and 1975, these researchers documented a tripling of the resistance rate for gentamicin.

Tobramycin, a still more recent antibiotic, had a similarly short life as a universally effective therapeutic agent. Between 1976 and 1977, just a few years after its introduction, tobramycin began to fail in treating infections caused by *Klebsiella, E. coli,* and *Serratia marcescens* in West Germany (in Frankfurt am Main), the southern United States, and Japan.

The newly introduced cephalosporins fared little better. *Pseudomonas* infections proved refractory to treatment, although *Klebsiella* was mercifully susceptible. In keeping with the general principle that resistance will be less likely for rarely used antibiotics than for commonly used ones, gentamicin proved effective against most of the bacteria for which it was prescribed. In contrast, penicillin remained effective against only 7 percent of *Bacteroides* microbes and 25 percent of the staph infections it used to wipe out routinely.

Other countries reported the same disturbing trend. In West Germany, between 1974 and 1978, resistance to gentamicin in strains like *Klebsiella, Proteus,* and *Pseudomonas* increased from two- to threefold. Even more alarming, researchers found that up to half of the isolated gram-negative bacteria could transfer their resistance to other species of bacteria. Throughout Europe hospital patients found their stays prolonged and hospital administrators saw patient death rates going up.

Similar patterns of resistance emerged for other bacteria that previously had been readily treated with common antibiotics. For instance, *Hemophilus influenzae,* a bacterium mistakenly named in 1920 as the cause of the influenza epidemic, has increasingly been found to be responsible for serious upper respiratory and middle ear infections. Infections that were easily treated with ampicillin prior to 1976 suddenly became resistant.

Between 1950 and 1970, a critical strain of *Hemophilus* (type b) responsible for a substantial proportion of childhood pneumonia and serious middle ear infections grew recalcitrant to tetracyclines in ever-increasing numbers. Respiratory infections caused by *H. influenzae* became increasingly resistant to this important antibiotic around 1971, and epiglottitis and meningitis became so in 1975.

It was not until June 1980 that the Center for Disease Control in Atlanta, Georgia, finally admitted that they had a serious problem. Triggered by the emergence of still another resistance pattern, this one to ampicillin, chief CDC epidemiologist Clyde Thornsberry finally admitted in that month that we were indeed facing a significant national problem.

Ampicillin-resistant *Hemophilus,* which is involved in such life-threatening infections as epiglottitis, cellulitis, pneumonia, and meningitis, as well as the previously discussed middle ear infections, had become an increasingly common cause of serious illness during the 1970s. Nurseries and pediatric intensive care institutions reported higher and higher rates of infection among newborns throughout this decade. In Washington, D.C., isolates of this organism with ampicillin resistance rose from 2 to 35 percent in just three years. Other cities, like Dallas, Huntsville, and Boston, reported similarly dramatic increases.

From 1976 to 1979, the overall rate of *Hemophilus* resistance to ampicillin went from 5 to 18 percent in the United States, causing widespread concern among pediatricians that this newly appreciated cause of newborn infections was going to go the way of staphylococcus and other groups of bacteria that acquired resistance to the major antibiotics. According to a Center for Disease Control survey of some thirty-eight states, the rate of increase in the isolation of resistant strains continues to be high. In

1980, some hospitals were reporting overall resistance as great as 38 percent. Striking increases in multiple antibiotic resistance in *Hemophilus* were noted between 1977 and 1982 in Great Britain.[5]

The sequelae of such infections can be extremely grave. One study cited in an editorial in the *Journal of Infectious Diseases* in November 1976 showed that among children surviving a *H. influenzae* infection, 6.5 percent are permanently incapacitated, 23.8 percent are left with a neurologic impairment, and 14 percent fail at school as a probable result of their bout with infection.

From a close look at a representative hospital it is possible to get a feeling for the extent of development of antibiotic resistance nationwide. The records of the North Carolina Baptist Hospital for the year 1976 reveal that during that entire period some of the bacterial species of the greatest health concern were resistant to commonly used antibiotics like ampicillin or carbenicillin.

Chloramphenicol remained the most effective antibiotic in this hospital's arsenal—and the most toxic. Indeed, instead of the broad range of antibiotics seemingly at the disposal of prescribing clinicians, most types of infections at North Carolina Baptist could only be expected to respond to one, or at most three antibiotics.

Problems of this magnitude proved to be more widespread than many epidemiologists thought. Soon it became apparent to virtually everyone that a constellation of factors had somehow turned the previous effectiveness of many key antibiotics on its head.

Just how much of a national problem antibiotic resistance is can only be estimated because of the lack of uniformity and relative paucity of records across the nation. Although such record keeping is now an almost universal requirement for hospital accreditation, underreporting is almost certainly the rule—and the true extent of the problem is yet to be measured, or felt. Its causes are nonetheless worthy of review.

---

[5] J. Philpott-Howard and J. D. Williams, "Increase in Antibiotic Resistance in *Hemophilus influenzae* in the United Kingdom since 1977: Report of Study Group," *British Medical Journal* 284, 1–4, 1982.

8

Inappropriate Use

One of the strongest claims of the drug manufacturers is that their products, when used rationally, have a remarkable degree of specificity in their germ-halting ability. With rare exception the ads for antibiotics urge the practitioner to perform routine sensitivity testing to determine if their product will, in fact, work against a particular strain of bacteria. This process is intended to determine the minimum inhibitory concentration (MIC) that will work against the offending pathogen. The most scrupulous researchers consider the MIC a minimum test in itself, and as a group have urged practitioners to use it wherever feasible.

The response to such an injunction has been less than overwhelming. In a single study of more than 194,000 different courses of antibiotic treatment at twenty different hospitals, over one third of the treatments were begun without a culture being performed to determine the sensitivity of the strains involved to

the antibiotic used. Where culturing was done the same researchers found that 39 percent of the patients never got antibiotics at all.[1]

Explaining this paradoxical finding proved difficult. However,
the authors of this careful study agreed that while it could be due
to an unusual streak of conservative practice at these hospitals, it
was equally likely to be the result of routine culturing irrespective
of need, or simply blind ignorance about how to read the results
of a culture. A more jaded view proposes that cultures are done
routinely *not* as an adjunct to rational medicine, but simply to
avoid the prospect of a later malpractice suit.

On any given day, from one fourth to one third of the patients
in American hospitals will receive an antibiotic. Only a minority
will have had their medication prescribed for a specific infection.
The rest will either have been treated prophylactically (i.e., in anticipation of infection) or been given a nonspecific, broad-spectrum treatment for a real, or suspected, infection. A survey done
at an Arizona hospital in 1981 revealed that fully 40 percent of
antibiotics used never should have been prescribed in the first
place, including 64 percent mistakenly used in an attempt to prevent infections.

Milton Silverman and Philip R. Lee, authors of *Pills, Profits
and Politics,* state the following on the issue of preventive treatment:

> The growing use of antibiotics to prevent infection has apparently
> been the principal reason for the rapid and indeed alarming in-
> crease in the prescribing of these drugs during the last few years.
> Some physicians justify this use on the basis that the risk is slight,
> the cost to the patient is usually not great, and the patient is
> pleased to see that his physician is doing something for him—and
> thus is not likely to turn to another physician. Evidence does not
> support such a belief. The best thing that might be said about
> the prophylactic use of antibiotics is that in most instances it is

[1] M. Shapiro et al., "Use of antimicrobial drugs in a general hospital. II.
Analysis of patterns of use," *Journal of Infectious Diseases,* 139: 698–711,
1979.

not clinically justifiable. It presents needless risks and causes unnecessary expense. At the worst, it may be fatal for the patient.[2]

While Silverman and Lee's classic exposé of the drug industry dramatically demonstrated the immediate consequences—in terms of adverse patient reactions and economic exploitation—of drug use, they largely underestimated the more subtle, long-term ecological ones. The health impact of changing patterns of microflora through injudicious use of antibiotics poses at least as great a problem for the long-term well-being of the populace as does the cost in misspent and misappropriated health dollars.

Using so-called broad-spectrum antibiotics as routine "first hits" for virtually any condition suspected of being of infectious origin was widely endorsed in the mid-1970s. And while the advocates of drugs like the tetracyclines or cephalosporins were quick to point out that such broad-swath approaches to wiping out an offending organism were intended solely as a first-line defense to be followed immediately by appropriate tests for specificity, their initial endorsement encouraged a generation of blind-treatment-minded physicians.

A representative quotation shows how even an enlightened approach can encourage the use of antibiotics without testing for specificity: "It might be said that the ultimate aim in chemotherapy could be to have two kinds of drugs; first, one would have a series of very broad-spectrum drugs, one of which would be used to initiate treatment of an infection before the pathogen had been identified. When the offending organism had been isolated, treatment would be changed at once to a 'secondary' drug, one with high activity against that specific organism."[3] In practice, the meaning of "at once" is subject to varying interpretations. All too often, the broad-spectrum antibiotic becomes the *only* treatment used.

The use of *combinations* of antibiotics to achieve a similar

[2] Milton Silverman and Philip R. Lee, *Pills, Profits and Politics* (University of California Press: Berkeley, 1974), p. 289.

[3] J. M. Hamilton-Miller and W. Brumfitt, "Whither the cephalosporins?" (editorial), *Journal of Infectious Diseases,* 130: 81–84, 1974.

broad spectrum of activity has generally been decried by concerned academic clinicians. While a few such combinations, such as the trimethoprim and sulfa drugs we have discussed earlier, may be justified, there is little support for the general use of two antibiotics simultaneously. Not only do many of the combinations that appear to work in laboratory bench tests (e.g., in vitro susceptibility tests) not work in practice, but interference between unrelated antibiotics has been observed—and, the encouragement of the simultaneous appearance of multiply resistant forms can be expected.

With these likelihoods in mind, it came as a surprise to see an advertisement in a 1980 edition of the *New England Journal of Medicine* advocating the use of a penicillin derivative called ticarcillin combined with gentamicin or tobramycin for treating a wide range of infections. The ad states in boldface on a separate page, "When Gram-negative infection threatens your cancer patient . . ." and then invites the clinician to use ticarcillin in combination with one of these other antibiotics. Again, it is only after reading the fine print that the reader learns that the only proven indication for the proffered combination is "against certain strains of *Pseudomonas aeruginosa*," for which "combination therapy has been successful, using full therapeutic dosages." Thus this combination is proven to work against only *one* gram-negative organism, not all!

In general clinical practice, however, combinations of antibiotics are commonly used for a variety of situations: when the cause of a particular patient's fever is unknown; when the risk of a second infection of the upper respiratory tract appears great (usually for a patient with a viral illness); when the clinician fears that bacteria may have entered the blood stream (for instance, after a transfusion where substantial amounts of blood are exchanged); after relatively simple "clean" surgery; after the discovery of a nonbacterial intestinal infection; or finally, in patients who have indwelling catheters that greatly increase the risk of infection.

As risk-laden as such situations may be for infection, there appears to be little or no indication for using combinations of antibiotics to try to prevent infection in *any* of these situations. In fact, in the words of H. F. Eichenwald and G. H. McCracken, Jr., of the University of Texas Health Center in Dallas, "Under these circumstances, combined antimicrobial therapy neither treats nor prevents infection; indeed, it is more likely that the risk of severe infectious problems is increased."[4]

Ironically, where a genuine need for finding two antibiotics that can work together has been uncovered—as in postoperative wounds where both aerobic and anaerobic bacteria commonly complicate therapy—little or no research has been done.

Many clinicians also advocate the use of broad-spectrum antibiotics routinely in the case of life-threatening disease. Of course the definition of when a disease comprises a risk to life or limb varies with the exigencies of the situation and the idiosyncratic views of the individual physician. A case in point is the advocacy position of Dr. P. E. Hermans of the Mayo Clinic. In this article[5] Dr. Hermans proposes that the clinicians concentrate on getting what he calls "broad antibiotic coverage" for any "seriously ill" patient through the routine use of broad-spectrum antibiotics.

Even though laboratory diagnostic aids now permit the rapid determination of the actual causative agents and their antimicrobial sensitivities, Hermans takes the clinicians' view that tests to select the most appropriate antibiotic "need not always be done." At the core of this conviction is the dangerously outdated notion that bacterial species are evolutionarily stable, having constant, predictable patterns of susceptibility to antibiotics. Hermans perpetuates this view by citing the belief that *Streptococcus* species, in his words, have "stable, predictable susceptibilities" to antimicrobial drugs. The outbreak of multiply resistant streptococcal infections in the nursery in Durban, South Africa, in 1977 (see Chapter 1) should have put the issue to rest permanently.

A further problem is that the proliferation of antibiotics and

---

[4] H. F. Eichenwald and G. H. McCracken, Jr., "Antimicrobial therapy in infants and children, Part I. Review of antimicrobial agents," *Journal of Pediatrics*, 93: 337–77, 1978.

[5] P. E. Hermans, "General Principles of Antimicrobial Therapy," *Mayo Clinic Proceedings*, 52: 603–10, 1977.

their inappropriate use was totally consistent with the economic needs of the drug industry. Increased uses for antibiotics that ignore major principles of clinical medicine have actually been encouraged by drug companies. One example is drug company advocacy of preemptive treatment before susceptibility testing. And advertising for antibiotics is notorious for frequent misrepresentation as well as the misleading suggestions for use seen above.

An instance of this type of abuse can be found in the advertising campaigns run during the critical period of the 1950s by the major drug companies. Many deceptive ads cloaked the actual identities of antibiotics. A representative journal of the times, called *Antibiotic Medicine and Clinical Therapy,* which had a circulation in the late 1950s of some 60,000 physicians and hospitals, carried ads that perpetuated the overuse of a time-honored drug by implying that it had novel properties in new forms. In one three-month period, from July to August 1958, this journal ran ten ads containing the product announcements of an antibiotic made by three major pharmaceutical firms, each represented by a different trade name, therapeutic use, and supposed composition. On closer inspection it was clear that the three companies, Bristol, Pfizer, and Lederle, were all advertising the same drug, tetracycline, disguised under three different brand names and three different formulations.

In reality, these companies held a virtual worldwide monopoly in production of tetracycline between 1952 and 1962, and cloaked its identity in every imaginable brand name variant to create the impression of clinical differences in indication and use. Thus, Bristol touted the presumptive benefits of Tetrex, its "sodium-free" tetracycline, Pfizer bragged about the unproven "superior absorption" to be found in its glucosamine-containing brand, Cosa, and Lederle announced the improved benefits to be gotten from its newest tetracycline addition, Achromycin with citric acid. The danger of this common proprietary practice is that it implied that varieties of the same product might have qualitatively different clinical effects.

The actual biological potencies of all these products were indistinguishable. But the implied variation perpetuated the belief in the medical establishment of a multiplicity of uses for tetracycline at the very time when, in fact, its uses should have been becoming increasingly circumscribed. Other medical literature of this period warned about cross-placental transfer of tetracycline and potential fetal damage from impaired calcium deposition in developing bones and teeth. Numerous reports expressed alarm about the increasing prevalence of antibiotic resistance as well.

A rather timid first step in the direction of restrictions on homologous antibiotics was taken in 1980 against a related product, erythromycin. Eli Lilly's Ilotycin (erythromycin estolate) was taken off the market in the first part of 1980 on evidence that it was neither superior to other formulations of erythromycin, nor as safe as the major products then on the market.

By 1975, drug companies such as Bristol Laboratories were capitalizing on the spread of penicillin-resistant staphylococcus to the community at large as a justification for pressing cloxacillin, under the brand name of their "new" penicillinase-resistant product Tegopen, on the market. Citing a 1977 review article in the *Mayo Clinic Proceedings,* the manufacturers urged practitioners to use "one of the penicillinase-resistant penicillins for all cases of gram-positive coccal infections before identification and susceptibility testing."

Such a lax policy flies in the face of standard susceptibility testing procedures established over ten years earlier. Major texts on antibiotics that discussed the therapeutic uses of antibiotics in hospital practice in the 1960s emphasized that such penicillins were appropriate only if a staphylococcus were *first* shown to be a penicillinase producer.

What had changed in the preceding ten years to justify *routine* use of cloxacillin (Tegopen)? First, it must be acknowledged that the proportion of staph infections resistant to penicillin did increase dramatically in the 1960s, particularly in infections outside of the hospital setting. But is this fact alone sufficient to warrant blanket use of cloxacillin?

The manufacturer's own fine print in a typical ad provides quite a different picture:

> Cloxacillin sodium is a compound that acts through a mechanism similar to that of methicillin against penicillin G-resistant staphylococci. Strains of staphylococci resistant to methicillin have

existed in nature and it is known that the number of these strains reported has been increasing. Such strains of staphylococci have been capable of producing serious disease, in some instances resulting in fatality. Because of this, there is concern that widespread use of the penicillinase-resistant penicillins may result in the appearance of an increasing number of staphylococcal strains which are resistant to these penicillins.

Brief Summary of Prescribing Information © *Bristol Laboratories 9/11/75 for Tegopen* (*Cloxacillin sodium*).

In other words, while the boldface ad advocates "blind" use of their product, the fine print embodies the spirit of conservative practice. This classic double message, i.e., "use our product without hesitation" and "use our product only with great caution," is typical of many drug company circulars containing prescribing information. Only here, the practice advocated, namely, the encouraged reflex to use Tegopen blindly, is acknowledged to contribute to the problem of antibiotic resistance that made the product necessary in the first place. In fact, were the drug company to be seriously concerned about the acknowledged "increasing number of resistant staphylococcal strains" it would have advocated avoiding blind use of their product, and urged routine prescription only *after* a susceptibility test had been performed.

In the 1980s, the use of broad-spectrum antibiotics prior to any characterization of the antibiotic susceptibility of the infectious agent is less justified than ever before. Drug companies, too, are recognizing the inherent contradictions between their stated objectives to provide means to reduce the incidence of difficult-to-treat infections and their wholesale push to get new varieties of old antibiotics into widespread circulation.

A case in point is the announcement in 1980 by Abbott Laboratories of a new automated susceptibility testing system. Called "MS-2," this system promises to afford clinicians sufficiently rapid turn around times on their specimen analyses so that treatment can be initiated with a proper antibiotic in less than two days, fully eighteen hours sooner than without the system.

Hospitals, too, are taking a belated but nonetheless more

enlightened view of their responsibility to offset the occurrence of hospital-acquired infections through early detection of changes in the strains and susceptibility patterns of bacteria on their wards. The University of Pennsylvania Hospital in Philadelphia, for instance, periodically reviews its base-line data over a twenty-six-week period to identify trends.

Large corporations have capitalized on this newfound responsibility. Bac-Data Systems in Clifton, New Jersey, provides over three hundred hospitals with a service that gives them trend information on the nature and type of infectious agents encountered in their hospital settings.

Of course, testing for antibiotic susceptibility becomes a moot issue if antibiotics are given when no infection is present at all. In fact, a disturbingly high proportion of antibiotics are prescribed in many American hospitals under just such circumstances, on the premise that a "prophylactic" or preventive effect will be gained. Theoretically, the belief that antibiotics could be used to offset the prospect of infection is not inconsistent with good medical practice—that is, *if* it works and *if* it is medically indicated.

Closer inspection of actual practice suggests, however, that prophylactic use of antibiotics often fails to follow such strict logic. In an age of litigation, some surgeons tend to use prophylactic treatment as part of the practice of defensive medicine. An obstetrician in Houston, Texas, for instance, routinely uses ampicillin as prophylactic treatment for each caesarean section she does—but only on her poor, publicly supported patients. Some of the logic here is impeccable: these patients as a group have an extremely high rate of postpartum infection of the uterus. But in the absence of controlled trials, the lurking suspicion remains that treatment is as much to compensate for poor staffing and perhaps minimize later legal problems as to offset the prospect of serious infection. Just having the "impression" of clinical efficacy is, of course, inadequate, and the fact that ampicillin then contaminates the mother's milk should be a serious consideration, since its presence can disrupt the infant's intestinal flora.

One way to measure the extent of what otherwise might be seen as simply an idiosyncratic practice, is to poll whole hospitals over a given period of time to determine what proportion of their dispensed drugs are devoted to antibiotic prophylaxis. Just such a study was done for the group of twenty hospitals in Pennsylvania cited at the beginning of this chapter.

At these mid-size hospitals, 31 percent of the antibiotics were prescribed in anticipation of infection, or at least so it seemed, since no indication of preexisting infection could be uncovered on the patients' charts. In following the patterns of prescribing practices, the researchers uncovered the startling fact that over sixty-two thousand doses of antibiotics were given to some five thousand hospitalized patients for nonexistent infections. As has been found elsewhere, prophylactic use comprises the worst category of misuse. Overall, from 50 to 65 percent of prophylactically prescribed antibiotics are found to be inappropriate in surveys like this one.

While some procedures do in fact justify prophylaxis, only rarely is there any indication to pretreat nonsurgical patients for protection against anticipated disease. One exception is the recent proposal to treat the family members of a child who has *Hemophilus influenzae* meningitis with the antibiotic rifampin as a precaution against getting this dread disease. The recently proven efficacy of a *H. influenzae* vaccine in protecting children from otitis media casts doubt on this approach. Three others include prophylactic treatment of cancer patients awaiting chemotherapy (to reduce the risk of *Pneumocystic carnii*), sustained treatment of asymptomatic women subject to recurrent urinary tract infections, and possibly, prophylaxis against traveler's diarrhea.

Most infectious disease specialists believe that antibiotic prophylaxis is justified only in those few instances in which adequate clinical trials have proven benefits from treatment; and then, only with very short courses of treatment or just a single dose. Such trials have shown that antibiotic treatment in anticipation of infection is appropriate for some forms of surgery, notably those done on the gastrointestinal tract and heart where infection is either very likely—or, as in the case of open heart surgery, dangerous in the extreme if it occurs. Some surgeons also advocate prophylaxis in hysterectomies, high-risk caesarean section, colorectal surgery, some forms of major vessel surgery, total hip replacement, and head and neck surgery. Such pretreatment used to be thought of as a means of sterilizing the blood, intestinal tract, or body cavity. Now, it is clear that antibiotic prophylaxis falls short of this goal.

When and if to give antibiotics prior to a surgical procedure was systematically reviewed by a panel of experts in the late 1970s under the sponsorship of the Veterans Administration. The practice of giving antibiotics during the immediate pre- or postsurgery period only rarely is done in accord with the guidelines for peer review proposed by these prestigious advisers. While the Veterans Administration guidelines severely limit the types of surgery where prophylaxis is allowed, over half of the antibiotics prescribed routinely go to uninfected surgical patients as prophylaxis for postsurgical complications. Of these patients fewer than half characteristically meet the specifications of the Veterans Administration panel.

Such errors cannot be considered innocent omissions since most prophylactic practices greatly increase the possibility of antibiotic resistance spreading to other organisms. For instance, the previously cited (p. 68) St. Paul–Ramsey Hospital epidemic was directly attributed to inappropriate uses of antibiotics as prophylactic measures.

While a few physicians and concerned administrators are taking pains to minimize the more flagrant examples of other abuses,[6] at one 125-bed Hawaiian hospital, the preexisting situation could only be described as grim. Here, clinicians routinely gave one quarter of all admitted patients antibiotics, among whom only 15 percent could expect to have gotten the correct prescription or right dosage regimen. Inappropriate use occurred in 85 percent of the cases.

Antibiotics are also consistently misused in the course of "normal" clinical practice in the mistaken belief that they can thwart the risk of infection in serious viral respiratory diseases, burns, trauma, or chronic diseases. Leading researchers Heinz Eichenwald and George McCracken believe otherwise. Without equivo-

[6] A relatively rare successful approach was published in 1974 in which temporary restrictions on antibiotics reduced total use significantly: J. E. McGowan and M. Finland, "Usage of antibiotics in general hospital: Effect of requiring justification," *Journal of Infectious Diseases,* 130: 165–68, 1974.

cation, these experts declared in the review cited previously that
". . . it has been repeatedly demonstrated that antibiotics do not
prevent infection when used for these purposes."

If antibiotics proved to be so ineffective in such widely divergent circumstances, what has been the rationale for using them so
extensively, particularly in surgery? Part of the answer rests with
the almost mythical belief in the ability of antibiotics to create
pathogen-free environments. But from the very first, indeed in
Fleming's original manuscript, the evidence was there that any individual antibiotic could only "clear" a portion of a mixed population of bacteria, leaving the others free to grow out.

Since Ignaz Semmelweis, who showed the importance of clean
hospital technique in the mid-nineteenth century, less assiduous
surgeons have relied on chemical crutches to achieve their hoped-
for success as measured by uninflamed suture lines, rapid drainage and closure of wounds, and an uncomplicated postoperative
course. Just as Lister's antiseptic solutions made war surgery possible (along with ether anesthesia), so antibiotics were expected
to make new forms of surgery a reality. And so they did—up to a
point. Open heart surgery, total hip replacements, and bowel
resections probably owe much of their success to antibiotics. But
the commonsensical notion that antibiotics could secure the cleanliness of any surgical field was as dangerous a myth as the belief
in the salubrious practice in Semmelweis' time of washing up
after rather than before delivering babies.

A procedure that I witnessed in 1957 illustrates the pitfalls of
the heightened expectations for prophylactic antibiotics in surgery
of that time. A young, obese woman was being operated on by a
new intern to remove an infected appendix. In the course of tying
off the highly inflamed appendix, he carelessly nicked it with a
scalpel and it ruptured into the abdominal cavity. The senior
surgeon who had previously ordered prophylactic penicillin now
ordered an immediate infusion of more penicillin into the per-
itoneal cavity. It was a case of too little too late—and a disastrous
surgical blunder. The woman later developed blood poisoning
and went into septic shock. Her infection proved so overwhelming
that she died within a week of the procedure.

In fact, it is not clear that, with the rare exception of specially prepared "islands" that are intentionally made bacteria-free for cancer patients, antimicrobial drugs can achieve the cleanliness so crucial to successful surgery. As a testament to this position, the author of the definitive handbook on antimicrobial therapy, Herbert L. Dupont, states categorically that (with the above-mentioned exception) "it is impossible to sterilize any area of the body by antimicrobial agents for significant periods of time."[7]

The experimental basis for even suggesting that antimicrobial agents reduce the rate of infection is surprisingly thin. The studies most frequently cited to demonstrate that antibiotics have helped reduce infection in certain surgical procedures, may more accurately depict diminishing rates of infection due to improvements in surgical technique.

In Dupont's antimicrobial "bible," the two principles that are most strongly advocated are (1) the antimicrobial agent has to be present during the procedure to have the desired beneficial effect and (2) prophylactic antibiotics should be used with surgery involving prosthetic devices as a means of preventing staphylococcal infections. Dupont emphasizes that prolonged, broad-spectrum antibiotic therapy only encourages the emergence and proliferation of antibiotic-resistant flora, with the resulting replacement of the native bacteria of the host.

One would think that with such a clear-cut injunction against the inappropriate use of antibiotics, prolonged postsurgery treatment would be the exception. Instead, study after study indicates that treatment continues well past the forty-eight hours recommended by the VA panel as the outside limit for antibiotic use after surgery. The consequence—more resistant organisms proliferating in the hospital with resulting increases in risk to patients. All too often, this development appears to be shrugged off as a necessary concomitant of defensive medicine.

Unfortunately, as we have seen, the microbial world does not stand still for human expectations. Only a few clinicians take a more enlightened view about broad-spectrum and prophylactic antibiotics. Dr. Maxwell Finland, writing in the prestigious *Post-*

---

[7] *Practical Antimicrobial Therapy* (Appleton-Century-Crofts: New York, 1978); p. 122.

graduate Medicine, has warned that to avoid antibiotic resistance only those antibiotics with the *narrowest* possible spectrum of antimicrobial activity should be used, and prophylactic use kept to an absolute minimum.[8] In lay terms, this means using a flyswatter and not an elephant gun to kill a fly, and only when the fly is in view.

Similar limitations have been voiced about combinations of antibiotics. The most representative and authoritative opinion on the use of combination drugs states that their routine use violates the widely held maxim that a combination of antibiotics should not be used unless therapeutic results with one of the drugs is known to be unsatisfactory.

An editorial in the July 8, 1978, *Lancet* conveyed the following expert consensus: "Meanwhile the unwanted effects of combined therapy—broader suppression of normal flora, increased risk of secondary infection caused by resistant organisms, obscured diagnosis, and adverse drug reactions—should temper our enthusiasm for antibiotic combinations."[9] In all, the most enlightened position regarding antibiotic use is that more ways of using existing agents should be sought before novel combinations are developed to "snow" the patient and thereby risk the further proliferation of multiply-resistant bacteria.

The provision of antibiotic care in anticipation of infection or in a blind attempt to suppress an existing one is thus obviously controversial. There are those who maintain that protective courses of treatment in anticipation of surgery or broad-spectrum treatments constitute nothing but the best preventative medicine. The fact that such treatment greatly increases the overall likelihood of hospital-acquired antibiotic-resistant infection is often of little concern to the surgeon or clinician who is treating a seriously ill or prospective surgical patient. In this sense, prophylaxis and anticipatory treatment exemplify one of the most critical issues of medical care: How should the individual practitioner

[8] "Superinfections in the antibiotic ear," *Postgraduate Medicine,* 54: 175–83, 1973.

[9] Anonymous, "Antibiotic antagonism and synergy," *Lancet,* 2: 80–82, 1978.

balance his or her treatment choices—as they affect the individual or as they affect the community?

This dilemma can often be found at the core of problems of inappropriate patient care and misuse of antibiotics, a theme struck by R. B. Sack, M.D., in a recent editorial in the *New England Journal of Medicine*. Sack described the intrinsic tension between the physician's loyalty to the patient and the needs of the community. Tracing the disastrous spread of antibiotic-resistant organisms and their resulting uncontrollable epidemic manifestations, Sack was among the first to recommend replacing antibiotics with "less ecologically disturbing techniques."[10]

Sack cites at least two examples where the attempt to use antibiotics to head off incipient infections in the individual posed grave risks to the community. The first was the attempt in Africa to use tetracycline treatment of as yet uninfected individuals as a means of controlling an outbreak of cholera. Within a few years virtually all of the cholera-producing strains in Tanzania were resistant to what had been one of the few relatively safe drugs that could control it. By 1978, Tanzania had experienced its fourth major epidemic, with little or no hope in sight for relief. Prophylaxis here was a complete disaster.

The second example is the as yet unproven use of a variety of tetracycline called minocycline, a drug that is generally believed to be capable of preventing gonorrhea infection if given before sexual relations. Whether it is desirable to extend this protection to a small portion of the sexually active population at the expense of the subsequent appearance of yet another antibiotic-resistant strain of gonorrhea was never adequately discussed before minocycline was made widely available for this purpose. The ultimate outcome of this experiment in medical microecology remains to be seen. But, if history is any guide the result is likely to prove disastrous.

What all this means is that physicians are going to have to rec-

[10] R. B. Sack, "Prophylactic Antibiotics? The Individual versus the Community," *New England Journal of Medicine*, 300: 1107–8, 1979.

ognize that the best possible treatment for the patient may not always be the best possible treatment for the hospital, the community, or the next generation of patients to come. "Blitzing" a seriously ill patient with broad-spectrum antibiotics to get that extra bit of insurance that an infection is controlled represents neither good medical practice nor sound clinical judgment if the long-term need for health protection of the community is factored in.

Even the use of an antibiotic with a seemingly fail-safe spectrum of activity (and recall that when they were first introduced, virtually every antibiotic had such a reputation) does not ensure that the next patient's infection will be effectively controlled. And the first failure may initiate the emergence of resistant organisms that jeopardize the hospital, or community as a whole.

Unfortunately the initial success that a physician invariably finds with the first use of a new antibiotic may encourage the blind adherence to that antibiotic for years to come, even as resistant organisms spread, and its effectiveness diminishes. Many readers probably know of doctors who still believe that penicillin is the wonder drug of all time, even though its effectiveness for certain common infections (e.g., staph), has been virtually destroyed through the emergence of antibiotic-resistant strains of previously susceptible organisms.

When, rarely, a powerful, broad-spectrum antibiotic is used appropriately in a life-threatening situation physicians can easily be lulled into believing that it should be tried in less exigent circumstances. Often ease of administration (oral versus injected routes) or decreased dosage schedules (two times a day instead of three or four) become the factors that sway the physician's choice for one antibiotic over another. When convenience dictates choice, the evolutionary consequences of that decision—and their ramifications for public health—are effectively ignored.

The testing ground for assessing the consequences of such behavior is the hospital. It is here that the most bacteria get the most exposure to the most antibiotics—and with these factors, the greatest opportunity to adapt, survive, evolve, and infect the next round of patients in a new, resistant form.

9

Getting Sick in the Hospital?

Since the work of Semmelweis in the mid-1800s, who described the unforeseen scope of the problem of puerperal fever in lying-in hospitals, the medical profession has known about the risk of hospital-acquired or "nosocomial"* infections.

Most patients go into a hospital with the presumption that they will have what is ailing them corrected. Few people think of a hospital as a place where they can get an illness that they didn't have before. But that is exactly what happens to a very large number of unsuspecting patients each year, and some of them even die of diseases they did not have when they entered the hospital.

A nosocomial infection is technically one that is independent of the illness or reason for a patient's initial hospitalization. For ex-

---

*Derived from the Greek *nosos* (relationship to disease) and *komein* (hospital).

ample, a person who is scheduled to undergo relatively simple elective surgery and then acquires a wound infection after his operation which prolongs hospitalization for several days to a week or longer has gotten a nosocomial infection. Similarly, an infant admitted to a hospital for a few days of medical evaluation for a congenital heart problem and then acquires a severe staphylococcal infection indirectly from another patient also has received a nosocomial infection. Nosocomial infections are of interest here because they are almost invariably caused by antibiotic-resistant bacteria.

The most common nosocomial infections are, in rank order, urinary tract infections, pulmonary infections, surgical wound infections, and septic phlebitis.

Overall, available evidence indicates that on the average approximately 3–5 percent of all patients admitted to hospitals in this country develop a nosocomial problem during the course of their hospitalization. Since there are about 30 million admissions to general hospitals per year, it can be estimated that between 900 thousand and 1.5 million hospital-acquired infections occur annually in the United States. Current statistics indicate about 1 in every 5,000 patients entering an American hospital will actually die of an infection contracted there. One researcher estimates that as many as 137,500 deaths per year could be caused or complicated by nosocomial infections of the lower respiratory tract alone.[1]

Hospitalization by itself does not necessarily predispose the patient to a nosocomial infection, but the hospitalized patient is often an "altered host" with enhanced susceptibility to infection because of either disease or therapy. Many cases are not recorded as instances of nosocomial infection, when they are in fact so caused.

One situation was described in the June 1980 issue of the *Western Journal of Medicine*. A fifty-three-year-old man suffering from mercury poisoning was brought to the University of Southern California Medical Center in Los Angeles. Nine days after

---

[1]M. La Force, "Hospital-Acquired Gram Negative Rod Pneumonias: An Overview," *American Journal of Medicine*, 70, 664–9, 1981.

admission, and in a debilitated state from his poisoning, he developed a chest infection. After a chest tube was inserted for drainage, he developed an antibiotic-resistant pneumonia and died shortly thereafter. The authors of the study concluded that while their patient "undoubtedly" died from nosocomial pneumonia, the contributing cause of his death was the prior exposure to mercury. Depending on the idiosyncrasies of a hospital's record system, the actual "cause of death" might be listed as either of the above.

Newborn infants are also particularly susceptible to infection, as are patients with impaired cellular or humoral defense mechanisms, and patients in whom the physical barriers against invasion by pathogens are breached, such as burn or postsurgical patients.

The advent of antibiotics brought the naïve belief that the final solution to the control of hospital infections was at hand. But by 1957, as the incidence of hospital infections rose sharply, it was clear that many hospitals were encountering major life-threatening situations caused by nosocomial disease. One study conducted in Seattle in 1957 showed that of 189 patients with staphylococcal infections, 100 had contracted and manifested them *in* the hospital and 32 others developed infection with the prevalent hospital strain within sixty days of discharge. Of the 189 infected patients, 24 died. Many of these deaths were in patients seriously ill from other causes, but the penicillin-resistant staphylococcal infection they acquired in the hospital played the key role in their demise.

As a result of the nosocomial problems experienced during the mid-1950s, the American Medical Association and the American Hospital Association recommended that the Joint Commission on Accreditation of Hospitals require every hospital to establish an infection control committee. The Commission enacted that requirement in 1958. Now, over twenty years later, it is recognized that these problems are far from solved. To cite but one instance, when the Food and Drug Administration restricted the routine use of hexachlorophene for washing newborn infants a few years ago, there was a dramatic upsurge of nosocomial staphylococcal problems in newborn nurseries. These outbreaks reemphasized the fact that most hospitals are still unable to effectively deal with the problem of nosocomial infections. Even a cursory look at the multiplicity of their possible causes shows just how complex an undertaking control has been.

An extraordinary diversity of modern-day developments and deficiencies contribute to hospital-acquired infections. These include (1) advances in surgery and adjunctive life-saving equipment and procedures like airway assist devices; (ironically, such innovations increase the infection risk while increasing the prospects of recovery from surgery because they introduce additional foreign material into the body and traumatize tissues); (2) inadequate education, surveillance, and control measures specifically directed to the prevention of nosocomial problems; (3) inaccuracy or insufficient specificity of laboratory diagnosis, due largely to poorly trained technicians; (4) lapses in preventive procedures, such as simple hand washing, owing to shortage of personnel and poor operative technique; and (5) the often reduced immunologic defenses of many debilitated, therapeutically treated, or chronically ill patients.

But most important of all, hospital infections appear to be linked to the development of resistant strains of microorganisms within the hospital environment itself. Proof of such indigenous development is dramatically found by examination of hospital waste systems. For example, waste effluents, from hospitals in the Gainesville, Florida, area contain a disturbingly high proportion of bacteria with hospital-acquired R factors when compared with the effluent from nonmedical facilities. And routes of easy cross-contamination for these bacteria in hospital wards were readily identified by the engineers who studied this problem.

But where does the infection begin? The most common hospital-acquired infections are those linked to the placement of catheters or other devices that pierce the skin of the patient and serve as a natural conduit for infectious organisms. Thus, urinary tract infections rank first among nosocomial diseases. Patients whose breathing is artificially supported because of impairment through congestive heart disease, prolonged anesthesia, or upper respiratory infections also often acquire secondary infections from their hospitalization. Surgical wounds, particularly those which follow long procedures in nonsterile areas, such as resection of the bowel, are particularly prone to infection. At the bottom of the list, but still a common cause of hospital infections, are those that result from bacteria which enter the venous blood system through catheters, particularly indwelling venous ones. Septic phlebitis, virtually unknown before the advent of extensive intravenous therapy, is now a common example of another antibiotic-resistant, nosocomial infection.

For many hospitals, the disease-causing organisms are "new" as well. In one of the most prestigious hospitals in Pennsylvania, about 15 percent of all nosocomial infections are caused by *Pseudomonas* bacteria. Many patients appear to harbor these persistent bacteria in their nasal passages, sputum, or urine, only to contaminate themselves following surgery. At this hospital, the water fountains, ice machines, soaps, and germicidal solutions were all found to be contaminated.

Closer examination of the statistics behind the nosocomial story reveals even more disturbing trends. Since July 1974, when its data system was revised to reflect the urgently growing need to detect the full extent of hospital-acquired—and most often antibiotic-resistant—infections the Center for Disease Control has been keeping records of the numbers of patients that acquire infections after they get to the hospital. For the decade of the 1970s (the National Nosocomial Infection Study was begun in 1970) this infection rate hovered between 3.4 and 3.5 percent, with slightly more patients likely to get infections at municipal or county hospitals than at community or teaching hospitals. Although this surveillance is urgently needed on a hospital-by-hospital basis, only eighty-three hospitals in thirty-one states reported during a characteristic period (1975–76).

Even among this relatively small sample, hospital-acquired infections were disturbingly common: of the 2,579,668 patients tabulated, 92,001, or just over 3.5 percent of all inpatients, were affected. Some of the more serious outcomes of infection, notably blood infection from a wound or other sites of infection, called secondary bacteremia, occurred in 4.4 percent of the hospitals reporting in the CDC's National Nosocomial Infection Study.[2]

These detailed statistics belie the disturbing fact that one third

[2] Morbidity and Mortality Weekly Report, U. S. Department of Health, Education and Welfare, Vol. 29 (46), November 18, 1977.

of *all* infections in hospitalized patients, including half of those contracted by leukemia patients, are nosocomial. (These numbers differ from those of the CDC because they include patients who enter a hospital with a preexisting infection, but who acquire a second or third after admission.) In aggregate, nosocomial infections affect 1.5 million patients each year, at an annual cost in excess of two billion dollars.[3] And if we may accept the statistics assembled by the National Nosocomial Infection Study in 1975, at least one municipal hospital exists where 10 percent of previously uninfected patients got infected during their stay (CDC NNIS Report for October 1977).

By recalling the pattern of use of antibiotics that was charted in the previous chapter, it becomes easier to understand one reason for these statistics: No one has yet devised a system to prevent at least one fourth of the patients at the typical American hospital from receiving antibiotics unnecessarily.

In an attempt to improve this picture, some hospitals have adopted a detailed surveillance program based on the series of eighteen guidelines issued by the Veterans Administration Ad Hoc Interdisciplinary Advisory Committee on Antimicrobial Drug Usage. A representative study was published in an article in the December 7, 1979 issue of the *Journal of the American Medical Association* based on the experience at Trinity Memorial Hospital in Cudahy, Wisconsin.

In reviewing these results, it is well to keep in mind that they are presented by the authors as the epitome of what can be done by a "genuine and active" peer review program, one that they believe exemplifies an ideal educational process rather than a policing function.

But is the 3.4 percent occurrence rate that they observed any more "acceptable" than is the 2–3 percent rate reported in the National Nosocomial Infection Study for similar hospitals? The

[3] These figures can be calculated from data presented in the Morbidity and Mortality Weekly Report for November 19, 1977, as follows: Patient days in 1973 totaled 11,084,850; at $102.44/day this equals $1,135,532,000, and multiplied by an inflation rate of 10–12 percent/year would give over $2,200,000,000 in 1980.

idea that three or four out of every one hundred patients entering a hospital can *expect* to get an infectious disease after they get there is mind-boggling! All the more so when you realize that we live in an age where reasonable aseptic and hygienic hospital routine is readily attainable with existing technology.

Even with surveillance operating, it is not unusual to find hospitals in which three fourths of the patients admitted to surgery still receive antibiotics prophylactically, far more than the proportion of surgeries where prophylaxis would be acceptable. And of these patients, a considerable proportion are likely to receive antibiotics longer than the recommended 72-hour maximum. Even more assiduous surveillance has resulted in pushing the figure of misapplied antibiotics, particulary in surgical practice, only a few percentage points lower.

Failures like these are not for want of effort to devise more effective means to control antibiotic usage. Intensive auditing of records, physician education, and the availability of special consultations have all been tried as means of lessening the burden that poor antibiotic practice puts on patient pocketbooks—and reducing hospital nosocomial statistics.

Of these three practices, only the most restrictive appears to make a difference. The authors of a 1979 study presented in the *Western Journal of Medicine* had to conclude that neither physician education nor making voluntary consultations available to prescribing physicians altered their use patterns for antibiotics. Auditing, the most noxious of the three approaches to physicians who are used to virtually total autonomy, produced marginal gains in rational treatment practices, but at the cost (one would think) of professional rapport.

The modest decline from the early 1970s to 1980 in the overall number of hospitalized patients given antibiotics (roughly from 40 to 30 percent) pales a bit when compared to the figures presented in Chapter 8 that show over a third of these treated patients were not tested for the type of infecting organism, or its sensitivity to the antibiotic prescribed. Nor do these data factor in the appearance of still other threats.

The latest event in the series of misfortunes that brings the problem of antibiotic-resistant bacteria to the fore in hospital settings is the discovery that staph organisms may become "tolerant" of antibiotics. The "tolerance" phenomenon, as we have seen in Chapter 4, is one where a bacterium withstands the assault of an antibacterial agent without actually degrading it or denying it entry through the cell wall.

Unlike community-acquired staph infections, the initial attempt to treat those acquired in the hospital with ampicillin or penicillin now routinely meets with failure. Addition of gentamicin, normally sufficient to wipe out all but the most hardy strains, likewise fails. It was at this point that clinicians should have realized that they were dealing with tolerant strains. But often, as the following case study shows, this recognition comes too late for effective remedial action.

In the Ohio State University Children's Hospital in 1979, forty-six patients were found to have staph infections, sixteen of which were discovered to be tolerant. Ten of these, from children with prematurity or leukemia, were the probable result of repeated hospitalizations. Six out of ten of these patients died, compared to six out of the remaining thirty patients in whom the infection was caused by a nontolerant, and hence much more readily treated organism. Obviously, tolerant strains should now be routinely considered a possible cause of dangerous nosocomial staph infections.

In spite of data like these, one argument frequently heard among infectious disease specialists is that an infection acquired at a hospital is simply part of the price one pays for quality care. In this view, a hospital-acquired infection is all the more benign because it happens at the right place at the right time: after all, you might ask, where would you rather get sick, one hundred miles from home, or in a spanking new hospital?

The answer might well be a hundred miles from home. At least there patients would not face the prospect of encountering bacteria that have already gone through a dozen or more patients and thereby increased in virulence, or survived in disinfectant pails, or contained a vast reservoir of resistance genes to antibiotics— typical situations encountered at hospitals throughout the country. As to the issue of harmlessness, consider the experience of just one major city hospital—Boston City Hospital.

In a study reported in 1979,[4] 645 patients with various infections were studied: 97 of these were found to have gotten their bacteria during their stay in the hospital. Of this number, 85 were studied in depth. Compared to patients with community-acquired infections, those who had nosocomial ones stayed two weeks longer on the average. A few individuals even acquired a second nosocomial infection while hospitalized. These latter patients stayed over a month (35.4 days) longer than the average of those whose infections were acquired in the community.

A complicating factor of almost every instance of nosocomial infection is that most of the bacteria that take up residence in hospital patients are already resistant to the antibiotics currently in use at the same facility. This fact should not be taken to imply that some other hospital is a preferred environment. Indeed, a major risk of this type of infection is to the patient who must be transferred to another hospital, often one committed to care of the chronically ill.

You might surmise that fewer of the patients who get sick *in* the hospital die there than do patients whose infections were acquired elsewhere. In fact, the relative risk of dying from infection can be as much as four times higher for patients who get their bacteria in the hospital than those who get sick outside. A disturbing study by Drs. Joseph Myclotte and Thomas Beam, Jr., from the Veterans Administration Medical Center in Buffalo, New York, suggests that hospital-acquired, antibiotic-resistant streptococcal infections are substantially more common—and serious— than is the same infection acquired in the community. Among sixty-two patients with pneumonia, Myclotte and Beam found that those who had acquired their pneumonia in the hospital were far more likely to die than were those patients who had gotten sick in the community. In fact, the nosocomial patients were three to four times more likely to succumb from pneumococcal bacteremia or pneumonia than were the patients in the community. Almost half of the hospital-acquired infections were preceded by a course of antibiotic treatment—compared to none of those acquired in the

[4] J. Freeman, B. A. Rosner, and J. E. McGowan, "Adverse Effects of Nosocomial Infection," *Journal of Infectious Diseases,* 140: 732–40, 1979.

community—suggesting a reason why the nosocomial infections
were so difficult to treat: the infecting organisms were resistant.
Fortunately, only 4 percent of patients who have nosocomial infections develop bacteremia, or blood poisoning, the highest-risk
nosocomial infection.

In spite of these figures, many physicians still regard nosocomial infections as a necessary evil, an accepted concomitant of
the risks of surgery or hospital stays in general. With hospital-
acquired infection rates averaging between 2 and 4 percent nationwide, one would think that nosocomial infections would not
have gotten off so lightly.

Why is it not more widely known that going into the hospital
can be bad for your health? At least one reason is that, until
recently, few doctors were aware that hospital-acquired infections
were either serious or that common.

Good medicolegal practice now requires that all relevant facts
pertaining to the risk of operative or hospital procedures be
revealed to the patient. Yet, the risk of hospital-acquired infection is rarely or never mentioned on the informed consent docu-
ments of most operative procedures.

In a sense, such an omission is understandable. After all, no
good surgeon would want to admit that in his or her practice up
to ten out of every hundred patients will develop a nosocomial
infection! Because the origins of nosocomial infections are often
laid at the feet of postoperative care, rather than at the initial
preparations for surgery or the procedure itself, such "discretion"
is perhaps excusable. But sometimes the surgeon's own complicity
results in the standard of care falling below the norm needed for
a salubrious outcome. A case in point from personal experience
might illustrate the matter.

A close colleague's wife entered a San Francisco hospital for a
caesarean operation. After the procedure she was placed in a
semiprivate room where another patient was recovering from her
surgery. This patient already had a postoperative infection that
did not respond to antibiotics. Two days after the operation, the
wife noticed swelling and redness around the stitches of the caesarean incision and notified the nurse. No action was taken for
another two days, leading to a suppurative staphylococcal infection requiring drainage and massive antibiotic treatment. She

could not nurse her baby and had to stay in the hospital an extra ten days. Left with a one-inch-wide scar as a reminder of her experience, she regrets the unresponsiveness of the staff, and is curiously grateful for antibiotics, which, while eventually curing her, were probably responsible for the high prevalence of antibiotic-resistant organisms in the first place.

Such instances illustrate more the dereliction and detached attitude all too common on some surgical wards than they do the failure of modern medicine. A recent survey of intensive care, postoperative suites revealed how commonly physicians moved from patient to patient without washing their hands. Such omissions point out the pressing need for some type of program for review of hospital practice, particularly in the use of the antibiotics that have so badly been abused in the past.

To their credit, more and more hospitals are instituting such programs. Unfortunately, these reviews are often directed at reducing hospital costs first, and lessening inappropriate use of antibiotics second. Because the prescription of an antibiotic still falls within the purview of a physician's discretionary judgment, it is often an "out of bounds" area for the kind of peer review that has become commonplace for experimental procedures, surgery, and complex care generally.

Following the promulgation of the Veterans Administration's guidelines for appropriate use of antibiotics, a personal inquiry to Dr. Paul Kotin, the principal author of this study, brought a most disheartened reply. I had asked Dr. Kotin whether any follow-up had been done to ensure that the guidelines suggested by the VA task force had been acknowledged and incorporated into working arrangements at the member hospitals nationally. Dr. Kotin replied that while he acknowledged the importance of this type of study, no real follow-up had been done, nor (astonishingly) did he or his committee know of a plan to do any!

To understand the causes for this discouraging situation, it is critical to understand that two phenomena were happening simultaneously. The first was the previously documented inexorable increase in antibiotic-resistant organisms. The second, and more critical, was the delay of federal regulatory agencies in responding expeditiously to the burgeoning threat these organisms posed.

While many infection control workers recognized the existence of major problems in reining in infections, until 1974 no systematic work was done in the United States to measure the effectiveness of various strategies to minimize the spread of infections, specifically those that arose in a hospital setting. Since the 1960s, the American Hospital Association and the Center for Disease Control have been urging hospitals to institute control measures. By the 1970s, thousands of hospitals all over the country had begun surveillance and infection control activities intended to stem the tide of nosocomial infectious disease.

At that time, the Joint Commission on Accreditation of Hospitals had reinstituted requirements for recording antibiotic prescribing practices, and many hospitals had voluntarily instituted peer review processes to ensure that some modicum of rationality accompanied prescribing practices.[5] But no one instituted a plan by which the overall effectiveness of these stratagems could be measured.

In 1974, however, investigators at the Center for Disease Control in Atlanta instituted a nationwide Study on the Efficacy of Nosocomial Infection Control (the SENIC project) to measure the outcomes of the application of these control and surveillance activities.

In May 1980, six years after the program began, the *American Journal of Epidemiology* published the first papers that signaled that this program was alive and well. Unfortunately, rather than the expected initial reports of efficacy that the medical profession had awaited, the papers in this special issue merely documented the methodology that had been put in place for evaluating the results. So in 1982, the medical profession and the general public still await actual reports on the results of the control programs that were supposedly instituted seven years ago.

Typical of these programs is one by Robert Haley and Richard Schattman, from the Center for Disease Control and the School of Public Health at the University of North Carolina at Chapel Hill, respectively. In a 1980 paper the authors reported on their

---

[5] By 1975 the American Hospital Association had distributed the 1974 edition of its manual on *Infection Control in the Hospital* to 20,500 physicians and hospitals; the CDC's *Outline for Surveillance and Control of Nosocomial Infections* was sent to a like number.

activities in soliciting data fully *four* years earlier. They surveyed virtually all U.S. hospitals and found infection surveillance and control programs in place among 3,145 of these or 87 percent of the hospitals responding to their inquiry, with about half reporting very active surveillance programs. (Figure 5.) Environmental monitoring has actually declined, while surveillance has shown a modest increase from 1970 to 1975. The rationale for concentrating on surveillance, in which the types of bacteria and their antibiotic resistance patterns are charted, rather than on environmental monitoring, was reported to be the poor returns from environmental monitoring as a means to detect future focuses of infection. An equally plausible reason is the dearth of trained epidemiologists to interpret and act on this exacting work.

Slightly less than two thirds of the hospitals reported that they had a physician or microbiologist supervising their infection control programs, 42 percent an infection control nurse. Although

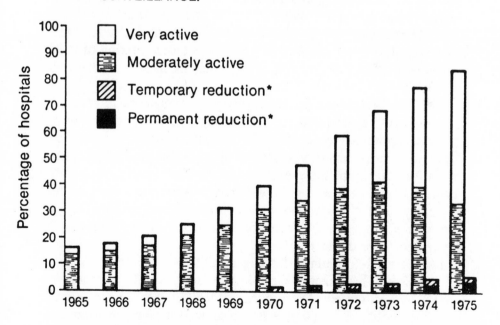

Figure 5. Levels of infection surveillance activities in 3543 short-term general hospitals with ≥50 beds in SENIC target population, 1965-75.
*Cumulative percentage.

three quarters of the hospitals reported that they had instituted
(under some goading one must assume) the practice of culturing
the environment for potentially contaminating organisms, a quarter of these reported that they had since discontinued this practice.

While the infection control movement that has emerged since
1970 is to be lauded, much ground still must be gained. CDC
bulletins and reports still record an alarming number of cases of
nosocomial infection. In the absence of a forceful antibiotic control program, surveillance of this epidemic is more window dress-
ing than cure.

Adding to this decline of what common sense would dictate as
a wise practice, the American Hospital Association issued a
"Statement on Microbiologic Sampling in the Hospital" by their
Committee on Infections Within Hospitals. Writing in the 1974
report of the National Nosocomial Infection Study, the AHA
concluded that routine microbiological environmental sampling
was both "unnecessary and wasteful." Such a finding, made fully
six years before the first national reports were released, would appear to be premature by any estimate. More likely, it was the
prospect of enforced, expensive environmental monitoring of hospitals that compelled the AHA to protect its members' financial
needs.

The AHA statement did acknowledge an obligation to conduct
retrospective reviews and surveillance *after* the occurrence of a
suspected nosocomial outbreak, in obvious disregard for the preventive purpose supposedly served by surveillance. Rather than
intensive follow-up, most experts believe that hospital infection
control should be designed to *anticipate* infection and head it off.
To carry out the AHA plan would be tantamount to abandoning
preventive strategies in favor of essentially useless "cleanup"
campaigns after the fact.

Dr. Calvin M. Kunin, a leading proponent of the rational use
of antibiotics, has taken a dim view of the medical community's
ability to institute effective programs to offset the dangerous epidemic of antibiotic resistance that is now sweeping the bacterial
world. As a member of various governmental advisory committees, he has strongly advocated the imposition of strict standards

for antibiotic use in hospitals throughout the United States. His pleas have generally fallen on deaf ears.

The intrinsic resistance of the medical community to outside control and "unnecessary" bureaucratic requirements effectively blocked the imposition of any regulations until the end of the 1970s, when a Joint Commission on the Accreditation of Hospitals ruled that antibiotic use must be audited in hospitals. Instead of the orderly process by which hospital record taking is generally accepted, Kunin found that this proposal was met with violent opposition.

The passive resistance to this proposal led to patterns of compliance that deluged hospital administrators and auditors in red tape and indecipherable records. It was as if physicians were using the old bureaucratic dodge of "giving them exactly what they ask for" as a means to ensnarl the whole system. Kunin, in an editorial in the *New England Journal of Medicine*[6] berated his colleagues for creating delays, paperwork, and frustration instead of the needed enlightenment for the rational use of antibiotics.

Among the points of contention for Kunin is the undue reliance on antibiotics with a purportedly broad range of effectiveness to control infections of unknown origin. As we have seen, the increasing reliance on so-called broad-spectrum antibiotics is encouraged by the industry itself, and by clinicians misplaced and often misguided concern about protecting their patients' welfare rather than in ensuring the retardation of the spread of antibiotic resistance.

In a related article that sparked heated controversy because of the implication that controls were necessary, Kunin stated that "we are dealing with a multifactorial phenomenon that requires an assessment of the constraints of practice."[7]

At that time, Kunin identified at least three factors that contribute to the flawed use of antibiotics: (1) the lack of integration of microbial services within a given hospital (e.g., between surgery,

---

[6] C. M. Kunin, "Antibiotic accountability," *New England Journal of Medicine,* 301: 380–81, 1979.

[7] C. M. Kunin, "Impact of infections and antibiotic use on medical care," *Annals of Internal Medicine,* 89: 716–17, 1978.

pediatrics, and obstetrical and gynecological services), (2) the inadequacy of physician training in the fundamentals of microbiology, and (3) the overwhelming expectations among physicians for efficacy of modern antibiotics—in a phrase, the belief in pharmacological infallibility. But are there simple solutions to this complex problem?

One generally recognized precaution is to ensure absolute cleanliness of the hands of hospital personnel, the most common source of infections that are acquired during hospital stays. Other less-well-known precautions are also feasible. Not only does the sensible process of screening hospital staff for unsuspected carriers of dangerous microbes reduce the frequency with which patients get infected, but as we saw earlier, simple aspects of antibiotic policy itself can be changed to reduce the prospect of contamination with resistant organisms.

A good example was recently reported from Gainesville, Florida. Here, a study of hospital workers showed that many were transmitting antibiotic-resistant infections to patients by touching patients and bedding with hands that served as a constant reservoir of infection. The dangerous spread of gram-negative organisms from the hands of pediatric nurses was found to be preventable by simply stopping use in the nursery of the antibiotics which selectively favored pathogenic strains. The authors of this key investigation recommended that restrictions of antibiotic use were a desirable means to control gram-negative colonization and infection.

Such rational judgment is to be lauded, but can it be extended to other settings in the absence of clear national priorities?

In spite of common acceptance of the idea that an increase in resistance among strains of bacteria is a direct result of antibiotic treatment, no one country really systematically tested this hypothesis until the mid-1970s. In a classic series of epidemiologic studies, Swedish researcher M. Jonsson conducted a before and after study of antibiotics' effects on patients' microbial populations, with particular regard to antibiotic resistance patterns. After a course of treatment with tetracycline or streptomycin, antibiotic resistance in *E. coli* increased by 50 percent. Patients who had entered the hospital for treatment of *Shigella* dysentery fared even worse. Initially, only 7 out of 35 were found on admission to carry *E. coli* bearing R factors. After antibiotic treatment, 29 of 35 had R factors. Jonsson concluded that inadequate antibiotic treatment readily enriches the proportion of resistant and R-factor-containing bacteria in the hospital. More critically, she recommended that to minimize this problem hospitals avoid tetracyclines, and restrict the use of sulfa, ampicillin, and erythromycin, a practice now being followed by some Swedish hospitals, but few if any American ones.

Even more disturbing is the realization that the problem of antibiotic resistance in the United States would now have little chance of being abated (as was successfully done in Sweden) through the implementation of a public policy directed solely at hospital prescription practices. The key to antibiotic resistance control, in my judgment, lies outside the purview of the hospital administrator. Unless two other realms of antibiotic use are simultaneously brought in line with hospital control, it is unlikely that any real progress will be made.

The lesser of these two remaining problem areas is the physician's office. Control of prescription practice here is so unlikely that one can only hope the example set by hospital practice will take hold elsewhere. Tort law presently provides little recourse to the public to sue practitioners whose prescription habits increase the risk of contracting an antibiotic-resistant infection. And successful suits of wrongful or negligent treatment with antibiotics are notable for their rarity, except for the most dramatic of reactions to penicillins or other allergenic drugs.

The final bulwark in the defense against effective antibiotic use resides in a much more unlikely place: the stockyard.

10

Antibiotics at the Feedlot

Nowhere is the flawed belief in the perfectability of nature more evident than in the human efforts toward domestication of animals. And among animals, the sine qua non of human eugenic ingenuity is said to be the steer. Raised on feedlots by the hundreds of millions all over the United States, the steer is fed a computerized diet of grains, roughage, and additives that increase its body mass at a remarkable rate. Some of these additives, like diethylstilbestrol, were expressly banned for their possible carcinogenic effects in humans, although at least 300,000 were still fed this illicit drug in 1980, five years after its use was suspended by the FDA. Surreptitious use of other quasisecret feed boosters and growth stimulants is said still to be common. We are concerned here with the key "stimulant," antibiotics.

It is not hard to understand the powerful motivations behind adding antibiotics to feed. With the annual cost of feed for 30,000 steers on a typical large lot reaching $5 million, the enor-

mous incentives to use any product that can increase—even marginally—the efficiency of conversion of feed into carcass weight is
obvious. And when that additive can be bought in bulk at a cost
of a few tenths of a cent per pound gained, any concern about
remote, second-order effects on populations miles away dims to
the point of extinction.

The issues behind the feed additive turmoil are classic in their
political ramifications, and almost impossibly complex in their
implications for health protection. Simply put, antibiotics are to
livestock production what the assembly line was to the auto industry: without it, production would stay at the level of a home
industry, communities would stay small and marginally well-off,
and overall "improvements" in production efficiency would be
measured in fractions of a percent rather than in terms of the
wholesale leaps made possible by economies of scale—or so the
advocates of antibiotic feed additives would have governmental
agencies believe.

In fact, the political issues go substantially beyond elementary
cost-benefit analysis. They envelop the whole gamut of factors
and consequences that come with wholesale shifts from small- to
large-scale farming, for no one denies that antibiotics are the key-
stone to mass production of livestock. As I will suggest here, the
trade-offs might be better seen in terms of second-order consequences (e.g., long-range health effects or community structure)
than first-order ones (e.g., productivity, beef costs, pork futures,
etc.). Weighing second-order consequences has a lot to do with
the attitudes that we foster toward community and overall public
health goals. But to appreciate these issues, it is necessary to
grasp just why the use of antibiotics has had such a hold on the
hog-producing, cattle-raising, and poultry-farming industries—or
more specifically, the agribusiness companies (pharmaceutical giants included) who would convert the livestock industry into one
giant mega-business.

In 1950, with cattle and hog production at an all-time high, experts placed hope for further improvements in production on bet-
tering their genetic stock. But additional help came from an unexpected corner—the pharmaceutical industry. Long over-inflated

in usefulness and oversold to the medical profession, antibiotics were available in substantial excess in the early 1950s. By 1960, production was increasing at 30 percent annually. Antibiotics had become a mass market commodity without a mass market.

The feedlot provided a ready market, as one large producer after another was sold on the often dramatic weight gains made possible by adding antibiotics routinely to their feed. Between 1950 and 1956, gains of nearly 5 percent over their previous norms were commonplace wherever hog or livestock density was high enough to have caused problems of diarrhea and other conditions related to crowding.

The existence of a glut of antibiotics combined with the exigencies of mass production and its concomitant losses, due to overcrowding, suggested a perfect solution: antibiotic additives at a few mils (tenths of a cent) per feeding created a chemical fix for poor animal husbandry. After all, the pharmaceutical detail men argued, all we are giving you is a cleaner animal. Feedlot producers accustomed to jamming steer, poultry, and hogs into unbelievably crowded conditions readily acquiesced to the self-evident: It made more sense economically to use antibiotics to do what would otherwise require a lot of hard work. Antibiotics provided, in the words of grower Henry Gilliam, "a substitute for management . . . a substitute of a chemical for hours of oversight."[1]

The rationale was clear enough. Thomas Jukes, codiscoverer of the antibiotic stimulant effect in feed, commented recently that "The usefulness of antibiotic feeding can be measured in the marketplace . . . I don't think we have so many cattle, pigs and chickens that we can afford to ignore feeding them by the most economical means."[2]

What this statement ignores is the distribution of livestock and its resulting incentive to rely on antibiotics. In the mid-1970s, 23 feedlot concerns controlled 14 percent of the market share with one-time capacity in excess of 50,000 head of steer per year.

[1] Quoted by George Anthan writing in the *Des Moines Register*, February 1, 1979.
[2] Quoted by Orville Schell writing in the *Co-Evolution Quarterly*, Winter 1980, "Wonder Drugs, Wonder Germs," pp. 96–107.

Fully half of all cattle were fattened on the 244 largest lots.[3] All rely on antibiotic supplements to their feed.

What brought us to this state of dependency?

Thirty years ago when antibiotics appeared to be a panacea for all of the ills that plagued a bacteria-ridden planet, it may have made sense to try this idea: If "clean" animals grew better than "dirty" ones—and certainly every stockman knew that—then why not lace livestock with antibiotics, particularly if these new wonder drugs were as safe for people as they were claimed to be? What harm could be done by simply adding a bit more to the diet of that steer in the yard?

Well, what was thought to be good medicine thirty years ago has not necessarily borne out to be good medicine today. If, as we now suspect, prophylactic treatment of humans with antibiotics is a direct invitation for the development and spread of resistance, similar exposures must be generating more of the same in the stockyard—or at least so one would think.

At issue is a very fundamental question: Just how much, if at all, does the nontherapeutic use of antibiotics for animals compromise the effectiveness of antibiotics in treating people? Obviously, if it is compromising human health, we should know about it.

HISTORY

The first real commercial use of antibiotics in animal feeds began remarkably early in the antibiotic era: By the end of the first decade of practical clinical use, Thomas H. Jukes, currently Professor in Residence in Medical Physics at the University of California, Berkeley, had reported that when chicks were fed rations containing a streptomyces culture, they grew dramatically faster. By the mid-1950s substantial numbers of livestock and chicken growers were experimenting with penicillin and other early antibi-

[3] Status of the Family Farm, 2nd Annual Report to Congress, Economic Statistics Service, Agriculture Economy Report No. 34, September 1979.

otics as seemingly miraculous new "growth factors." The most dramatic results came with the advent of intensive rearing practices in which animals were raised in ever more confined quarters. There the risk of epidemics or chronic infections normally cut back on any gains made by increased efficiency of production, until antibiotics came along. Antibiotics seemed to make it possible to raise more animals in less space, using less feed, and over a shorter period than through the use of conventional methods.

The actual tonnage of antibiotics used in animal feeds has increased dramatically since the 1960s. In 1960, livestock producers used only about 1 million pounds as a feed additive. By 1985, they used over 17 million pounds. In 1980, 75 percent of all cattle, 90 percent of swine and veal calves, 50 percent of all sheep, and virtually all poultry received antibiotics at some time during their production. The actual number of farmers who rely heavily on antibiotics has grown proportionately. In a representative survey done in the 1970s, 62 percent of Missouri farmers responding to a questionnaire acknowledged that they depended on antibiotics to a significant degree. Major producers with net incomes of $100,000 or more annually, relied on antibiotics the most, with almost 80 percent dependent on antibiotics for maintaining their rearing practices.

By 1974, nonmedical uses of antibiotics, principally in animal husbandry, comprised three fourths of all production—8.2 million pounds out of a total of 12.6 million. By the end of the decade nonmedical use had almost doubled, making agriculture applications the largest share of the traditional (e.g., penicillin/ tetracycline) market. In 1979, American pharmaceutical manufacturers sold almost a quarter billion dollars' worth ($243 M) of antibiotics for animal use alone. By that year, four major antibiotic groups had been approved by the FDA for use singly or in combination as feedstuff additives: *penicillin*, used principally in poultry and to a lesser extent in swine; *tetracyclines*, used in all food animals; *sulfa drugs*, used primarily in swine; and *nitrofurans*, used in chickens and turkeys, and to a lesser extent in swine.

The first concerns about health effects were voiced almost as an afterthought. In 1955, a group of scientists convened a conference under the auspices of the National Academy of Science in Washington, D.C., to discuss the economic aspects of the problem, and, belatedly, invited Dr. Maxwell Finland of Boston City Hospital[4] to speak about the possible effects on human health. The lines were drawn, with Finland and his co-workers warning about the long-term adverse health effects, and Thomas Jukes, one of the cofounders of the principle of using antibiotic supplements (with E. L. Robert Stokstad), steadfastly defending their use.

In March 1960, a joint Agricultural and Medical Research Council Committee (named the Netherthorpe Committee, after its chairperson) was established in Great Britain expressly to examine the possible human health consequences of antibiotic use. Like the first NAS committee, this group spent a significant portion of its research documenting the cost effectiveness and positive risk-benefit factors associated with antibiotic use.

These narrow-sighted findings held sway until 1968, when the Swann Committee was jointly appointed by the Minister of Agriculture, Fisheries and Food and the Minister of Health. The event that triggered this historic collaboration was an epidemic of *Salmonella* diarrhea from 1964 to 1966 in *both* calves and people, an outbreak in which an appreciable number of the human *Salmonella* strains (22 percent) showed the same pattern of antibiotic resistance found in the calves' *Salmonella*. In 1969, the Committee submitted its provisional findings, recommending banning any antibiotic that was commonly used in human therapy and requiring a veterinarian's prescription for any other antibiotic intended for use as a feed supplement for livestock or calves. (Figure 6.)

In part because of evidence indicating likely extension of other animal salmonellosis epidemics, the Swann Committee in March 1971 further recommended that all antibiotics be banned from use in the feed of pigs and chickens, except on veterinary prescription. In short order, Britain's lead was followed by the

---

[4] In a recent review of his experience at Boston City Hospital, Finland was substantially more conservative about the link between antibiotics on the farm and resistant infections in the hospital.

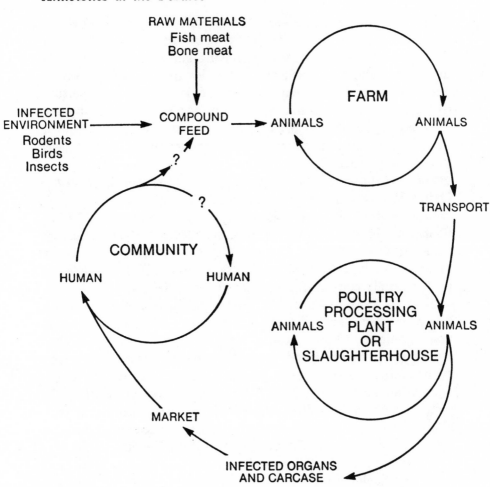

Figure 6. Chain of Salmonella transmission.

Netherlands, West Germany, Norway, Sweden, and Denmark. Opponents of these requirements were quick to point out that no reported incident existed at the time of their recommendation (1970–71) where pigs or chickens had served as the epicenter of a human infection. The simultaneous outbreak in calves and people observed some five years earlier could have been a fluke occurrence. Elsewhere, the caution many felt was so lacking from the British policy group was abundantly in evidence.

In the United States a report prepared at about the time the Swann Committee began its deliberations was submitted to the FDA in May 1966. While no "smoking gun" has been found in the United States to implicate antibiotics in direct outbreaks of human disease, the evidence in the late 1960s appeared persuasive concerning the likelihood of such an event. The committee therefore urged a series of cautionary moves, only one of which, the direct banning of antibiotics as a preservative of meat, was actually implemented.

Figure 7 shows the increased prevalence of salmonellosis in the United States for the period 1950 to 1979.

In a pattern that has consistently plagued those opposed to antibiotic use in animal feed, the FDA solicited the assistance of the National Research Council of the National Academy of Sciences rather than rely on its own regulatory authority. In June 1967 the NAS dutifully convened yet another conference and published its findings in 1969. Two papers in particular, one by Dr. E. H. Kampelmacher, Head of the Laboratory for Zoonoses of the National Institute of Public Health in the Netherlands, and the other by Dr. D. H. Smith, Chief of the Division of Infectious Diseases at the Children's Hospital in Boston, dismissed the use of antibiotics in animals as a source of human infection. As responsible public health officials, both experts noted the occurrence of precisely the same strains of antibiotic-resistant bacteria in humans and animals, but inexplicably rejected that the animal-derived strains could be causing human disease.

For Kampelmacher, the fact that mortality had not gone up appreciably in the Netherlands at the same time that antibiotic-resistant *Salmonella* were being isolated made the problem more of academic interest than of real public health concern. Smith put the entire blame of the emergence and spread of antibiotic-resistant organisms on the hospital.

Once more, in the spring of 1970, the Commissioner of the FDA, Dr. Charles C. Edwards, appointed a Task Force on the Use of Antibiotics in Animal Feeds. The Task Force, after visiting with members of the Swann Committee and convening a series of conferences and meetings in this country, issued its findings in January 1972, almost exactly a year after the Swann

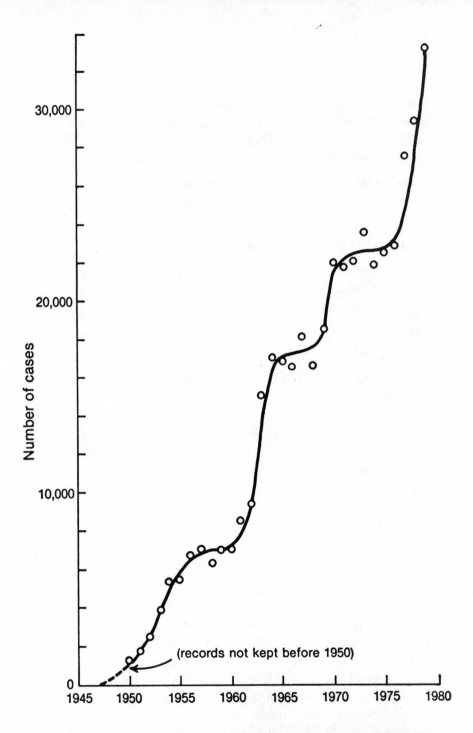

Figure 7. Increasing prevalence of salmonellosis in the United States 1950 – 79. Each reported case is estimated by the Center for Disease Control to represent approximately 100 cases that go unreported.

Report. On February 1, 1972, a provisional policy statement of antibiotic and sulfonamide drugs in animal feeds was published in the Federal Register. The Task Force drew five conclusions on the possible health risks of antibiotic use:

1. that the use of antibiotics, especially in subtherapeutic amounts, favors the selection of R-factor-bearing bacteria

2. that animals so treated may serve as a reservoir of antibiotic-resistant organisms that cause human disease

3. that the occurrence of multiresistant R-factor-bearing bacteria in animals has increased in direct relationship to the use of antibiotics in feed

4. that such resistant bacteria have been found on meat and meat products

5. that there has been an increase in antibiotic-resistant bacteria in human populations

Such evidence would seem to provide more than ample cause for restrictive action. Students of the law might readily see a case for "probable cause" in linking antibiotic-resistant *Salmonella* to human diarrheal disease, but the industry critics would have none of it. In a lengthy rebuttal to these well-reasoned conclusions, J. S. Kiser of the American Cyanamid Company's Agricultural Division, itself a major producer of antibiotics for animal feed, offered the following almost sophist arguments: Since bacteria don't have fingerprints, there was no way to link the admitted reservoir of antibiotic-resistant bacteria in animals to any appreciable outbreak of human disease. Even where the serotypes or antibiotic resistance profiles were identical (and there were cases to match this test), Kiser reasoned that it was impossible to link any *specific* bacterium in humans with an animal origin.

Kiser was joined in this line of argument by industry representatives and the American Society of Animal Science, all of whom followed the undeniable but nonetheless specious reasoning that held out for "definitive" proof.

Faced with a coordinated and sustained attack, the FDA issued an amended policy in the Federal Register of April 20, 1973, that acknowledged the economic value of antibiotic additives to animal feeds, emphasized that the case for human health risks could only be made for *Salmonella,* and provided industry with the obligation to demonstrate that their products did not increase the quantity, number of organisms "shed," or duration for such shedding of *Salmonella* from the animals fed their products.

In a particularly bold move, the FDA then mandated that any manufacturer who wished to maintain one of its products on the market had to show its safety with regard to these factors within a year. Companies like American Cyanamid, whose chief products were chlortetracycline (Aureomycin) and sulfamethazine (Sulmet), performed exhaustive tests to demonstrate that it was impossible to show that increases in the amount of antibiotic-resistant bacteria that were shed or produced were a direct result of using their products.

In 1974, the FDA had to swallow its edict, and a rather enormous defeat, particularly since it did not define what would constitute grounds for banning a specific product. One year later, this agency reluctantly asked its National Advisory Committee to reexamine all of the information and come up with a recommendation for policy alternatives by the next year.

EVIDENCE

Just what evidence can we reasonably expect them to have reviewed? In 1974, data were on hand for animal-to-human transfer. In Scotland, precise records of the types of *Salmonella* bacteria that cause disease are kept by the Scottish Salmonella Reference Laboratory. These records show that between 1974 and 1976, 137 different kinds of *Salmonella* caused disease in humans and cattle, but only four kinds were responsible for 52 percent of the epidemics that occurred over the two-year period.

Each of these four strains of *Salmonella* was commonly isolated from cattle—and each caused considerable outbreaks in humans. Without question, this study showed that cattle can be major reservoirs of infection for other animals—and people.[5]

In the years between 1973 and 1975, a second myth was being shattered: that feeding antibiotics to animals known to be major sources of human *Salmonella* food poisoning does not increase the risk of cross-infection. In systematic studies done over a six-year period, two researchers, Dr. H. W. Smith and Dr. J. F. Tucher, at the Houghton Poultry Research Station in Huntingdon, England, showed that feeding chickens a variety of antibiotics, including the widely used human antimicrobials lincomycin and bacitracin, altered their microflora dramatically and actually increased their colonization with *Salmonella* species!

While this effect was less striking with bacitracin than with the other antibiotics, the implications of the result were so grave that the authors concluded that the general use of antibiotics in feed additives should be discouraged. If feeds were to be supplemented they recommended using agents like sodium arsenilate, which actually discourages such colonization. But, of course, arsenic, a human carcinogen, is not likely to prove to be the most salubrious food additive should any residues accumulate in chicken meat.

Thus, it is hard to imagine that by 1975, there was *anyone* who did not at least believe that the *potential* for a major problem existed. But only a small group of scientists were firmly convinced that the pattern of antibiotic usage on feedlots was contraindicated, scientifically or in the interests of protecting public health.

During the period 1975–76, the almost simultaneous publication of at least two significant articles in the medical literature should have tipped the balance in favor of recognizing the need for curtailing antibiotic supplements to animal feeds. The first, by C. H. L. Howells and D. H. M. Joynson, appeared in the journal *Lancet* in 1975. Howells and Joynson showed that the animal feeds themselves are contaminated with antibiotic-resistant *Salmonella* and *E. coli*. These researchers emphasized the plausi-

[5] E. Barker, D. C. Old, and J. C. M. Sharp, "Phage type/biotype groups of *Salmonella typhimurium* in Scotland, 1974–1976," *Journal of Hygiene, Cambridge*, 84: 115–25, 1980.

bility that links between contaminated feeds, contaminated meat, and hospital patient diets could lead to the spread of antibiotic-resistant bacteria into susceptible human populations.

The second major article was written in the *New England Journal of Medicine* in 1976 by American researchers S. B. Levy, G. B. Fitzgerald, and A. B. Macone. They documented a clear and unequivocal transfer of antibiotic-resistant bacteria from chickens to farmers some five to six months after introducing antibiotic supplemented feed. This latter group of researchers was sufficiently convinced of the persuasiveness of its findings to urge against the unqualified and unlimited use of drug feeds in animal husbandry, and to appeal for a reevaluation of this practice.

Mass production in the feedlot augured badly for the kind of individualized treatment based on accurate diagnosis and susceptibility testing that competent veterinarians recognize as the hallmarks of good antibiotic practice. The 17.5 pounds of antibiotics currently fed to animals thus perpetuate a pattern of irrational practice that has stirred debate but little effective action. As Peter Singer and Jim Mason point out in their book, *Animal Factories* (Crown Publishers: New York, 1980), special "health programs" had been routinely used throughout the 1970s, as a kind of blitzkrieg of chemicals to stave off the likelihood of mass epidemics fostered by the incredible density achieved by livestock rearing practices.

The proof that such antibiotic practice is unneeded comes from experimental studies that pointedly demonstrate the total absence of a growth-promoting effect of antibiotics given to germ-free animals—or even for those that are raised with the bare minimum of good husbandry practices and sanitation. In light of the evidence, the bulk of this practice could be seen simply as a convenient chemical sop to offset poor animal husbandry practices. By 1976, the stage was thus set for regulatory action.

REGULATORY ACTION

On February 1, 1977, the FDA's National Advisory Food and Drug Committee concluded that antibiotics used to treat people should be eliminated from animal feeds. With this kind of support, the FDA prepared preliminary policy options that included the banning of antibiotics intended for human use as animal feed supplements. But implementation of any of these options was postponed pending review by the new FDA commissioner. His conclusions were not long in coming.

On April 15, 1977, within two weeks of taking office, the newly confirmed commissioner Donald Kennedy issued a "talk letter" to government agencies, health departments, and industry informing them of his intention to proscribe the use of penicillin and tetracycline in animal feeds. With the FDA order, antibiotics intended for animal consumption would have to be treated as if they were prescription drugs, the same approach used by the Swann Committee. If farmers, dairy producers, and stockyard operators wished to use these antibiotics, they had to solicit a prescription from a veterinarian. On the assumption that such prescriptions would only be ordered in the face of *existing disease,* this political solution appeared to spell the end of antibiotic feed supplementation with human-use antibiotics.

If there was any confusion about the FDA's ultimate intent, it was quickly dispelled by the chilling words at the end of the letter:

> These actions should be viewed as a first step toward FDA's ultimate goal of eliminating, to the extent possible, the nontherapeutic use in animals of any drugs intended to treat disease in man.

In Kennedy's judgment, the economic benefits so readily demonstrated by industry simply did not outweigh the potential risks to human health. Many policy advisers then in public health agencies, like myself, applauded this unprecedented forthrightness. In California, I drafted a letter of support for the commissioner's findings, citing the weight of medical literature reviewed above, and urging their formal adoption. The letter was signed by then Director of Health Jerome Lackner, M.D.

With hindsight, many have felt that Kennedy should have

waited until more definitive data were available on which to project the human risks. As it was, strict constructionists could still show that the risks were largely theoretical, and Kennedy was forced to acknowledge that he could not point to any specific instance in which human disease was actually rendered more difficult to treat because of drug-resistant organisms directly acquired from livestock or poultry. At best, Kennedy could only emphasize that even if such cross-infections were occurring commonly, they would not be detected by the surveillance systems then in place. He underscored the commonality of the microorganisms in human and animal ecosystems, stating that "The evidence indicates that enteric microorganisms in animals and man, their R plasmids, and human pathogens form a linked ecosystem of their own in which action at any one point can affect every other."

This eloquent but arcane statement merely served to enrage the livestock producers and their drug company colleagues. Lobbying intensively, representatives of these interest groups were successful in getting Congress to ask Kennedy for yet another reading!

Congress sent Kennedy's proposed regulations to the National Research Council of the National Academy of Sciences for review. In April 1980, the NRC concluded that data about the possible human health effects of antibiotic feed additives simply could not be evaluated. In the words of this prestigious eleven-member panel, "insurmountable technical difficulties" stood in the way of a precise rendering of judgment regarding the safety of drug additives.

From the National Research Council's scientific viewpoint, there simply were no adequate epidemiologic studies to show that a plausible health hazard was in fact a real one. Existing studies, they maintained, neither proved nor disproved the link between antibiotic use, resistant bacteria, and human disease. Moreover, it appeared to the NRC to be impossible to separate the resistant organisms that might be generated from the therapeutic (and hence justified) use of antibiotics to treat human disease from the non- or subtherapeutic uses in animals. Among the factors that the authors cited as being more likely to contribute to the acknowledged spread of antibiotic resistance, the NRC singled out the use of antibiotics like tetracycline to treat acne vulgaris in teenagers.

What is really going on here? Do the consequences of the use of antibiotics really just blur into the overall risks we incur by using antibiotics generally?

ARGUMENTS

A closer look at the arguments of the key participants is illuminating. One of these participants in the animal feed situation has been a group formed at the Ames Iowa State University called the Council for Agricultural Science and Technology (CAST). This group had been asked to provide input to the FDA's decision-making procedures on antibiotic supplements for animal feeds. Its report to FDA commissioner Donald Kennedy was intended to provide scientific background to this controversial issue.

In December 1978, however, six of its members wrote a pointed letter of protest stating that the draft of the final report omitted unfavorable evidence showing that drugs in animal feed were *not* as safe as alleged. In all, seven members of the panel believed that the final report failed to give adequate weight to the views of the microbiologists on the panel. Some of the information given the group for review in November was apparently ignored, or worse hidden, in the rush to get the final proceedings into print.

Among the most outspoken critics was Dr. Richard P. Novick, chief of the Department of Plasmid Biology in New York State's Department of Public Health Research Institute. On June 1, 1979, in a letter to *Science,* Novick wrote that "I have strong misgivings about the waste of one of our most valuable medical resources as a cover for substandard practices in the rearing of livestock, even if it is sometimes effective and saves the time, money and effort needed for decent animal management."[6]

[6] Richard P. Novick, "Antibiotics: Use in animal feed" (letter), *Science,* 204: 908, 1979.

In 1980, the CAST group, representing some twenty-five different agricultural science societies, endorsed the use of nine different antibiotics for use in cattle: bacitracin, bacitracin methylene disalicylate, zinc bacitracin, chlortetracycline, aureomycin, erythromycin, neomycin, oxytetracycline, and tylosin. This list is more notable for what it leaves out than for what it includes.

Penicillin is recognized as the backbone of much of the livestock industry's reliance on antibiotics, so excluding it is at least a step in the right direction. But what about the remaining antibiotics? Might not they also pose indirect risks to public health?

The evidence suggests that they do. First, it must be observed that other nations have not shared our reticence to proscribe antibiotic feed supplements. The Japanese, the Czechs, and the British have long recognized that animals can serve as reservoirs of potentially dangerous drug-resistant bacteria. And, contamination of one segment of the ecosystem virtually ensures contamination of all others. For instance, in an article by three Japanese scientists it is reported that over one fifth of all the pigeons that they examined (domestic or wild) were found to contain a majority of multiply resistant *E. coli*. Since one mainstay of these pigeons' diet was feedlot corn and debris, the fact that most bore R factors for at least three major antibiotics in use in treating human disease (chloramphenicol, streptomycin, and tetracycline) made them potential vectors for carrying germs or genes with antibiotic-resistant instruction from animals to humans.

If such spread is true or even likely, then why the reluctance to accept the probability of risk? Part of the answer comes from a line of argument developed by Kenny S. Crump in the OTA's *Drugs in Livestock Feed* issued in June 1979. In this paper Crump, a Professor of Mathematics and Statistics at Louisiana Technical University, states that "A high level of ignorance exists with regard to the quantitative aspects of [the] population dynamics . . . [of] the transfer of resistant bacteria and their R-plasmids from animals to humans . . ."[7]

It is precisely this kind of academic reticence that throws a

---

[7] Kenny S. Crump, "Estimating Human Risks from Drug Feed Additives," *Drugs in Livestock Feed*, Vol. II, Background Papers, Office of Technology Assistance, June 1979.

cramp into effective regulatory action. If even the experts are confused, the argument goes, then how can officials be expected to act? A closer reading of Crump's work, however, provides ample basis for action. He points out the following, for example:

1. It is known that long-term subtherapeutic feeding of antibiotics causes an increase in the proportion of resistant organisms in the intestinal tracts of treated animals.

2. Even feeding just one antibiotic can lead to the appearance of multiple resistance to a broad spectrum of antibiotics.

3. Once in the animal's intestinal tract, antibiotic-resistant bacteria can thrive, even after the use of the drug is discontinued.

4. The genes that carry this resistance, when present on R factors, can theoretically transfer it from nonpathogenic *E. coli* in animals to human pathogens.

5. The origin of the genes or bacteria is immaterial in conferring antibiotic resistance.

6. The normal course of animal-human contact opens numerous possible routes for spread of resistance genes, including direct contact, contact with food, and contact with feces or sewage in the environment.

7. The ability of some bacteria to cause disease is carried on R factors.

8. The treatment of some human diseases is being compromised by increasing resistance of pathogens to antibiotics.

Professor Crump calculated that approximately 2,025 Americans each year contract a serious invasive infection from just one antibiotic-resistant bacterium alone, *Salmonella;* and, for these people effective treatment is compromised by that bacterium's resistance. It was also evident to Professor Crump that the rapid increase of broad-spectrum antibiotic resistance in *Salmonella* probably means that it is going to become very difficult to treat invasive *Salmonella* effectively with antibiotics in the future. But

Crump's scientific caution prevented him from taking the argument to its logical conclusion,[8] namely, that these associations add up to a significant potential public health hazard. The final invitation to misunderstanding comes when Crump admits that it is impossible to know the exact rate at which R plasmids are transferred from animals to humans.

Crump's most compelling argument is thus easily lost to policy makers who may be told by interpreters of these data of the uncertainties, rather than the overall argument advanced by this careful statistician. In his view, "the existence of an enormous pool of R-plasmids such as now exists in the animal population, together with the ability of an R-plasmid to be promiscuously transferred among bacterial species must be regarded as a serious threat to the integrity of the therapeutic value of antibiotics in the treatment of human diseases . . . It could only be described as foolhardy not to curtail any unnecessary practice that contributes to the enlargement or maintenance of the R-plasmid pool in animals . . ."[9] (which of course is what we do every time we feed animals antibiotics).

In spite of such seemingly compelling arguments, the NRC saw fit to dismiss the thinking of the OTA Task Force as mere theorizing. To reach this conclusion, the NRC must also have dismissed the findings of Dr. Novick. His contribution to the OTA study did not mince words: Novick states unequivocally that "It must be noted at the outset that there is a vast body of data that, taken as a whole, demonstrates beyond any reasonable doubt that subtherapeutic antibiotic feeding to livestock promotes the emergence and maintains the prevalence of multiply resistant coliforms and *Salmonella* and that these spread in large numbers to the

[8] In the body of Professor Crump's report (ibid., pp. 65 and 66) we find two conflicting statements that could readily be misconstrued by the NRC: First, Crump states that we should keep in mind "that there is considerable evidence to implicate use of antibiotics in food-producing animals as the source of the bulk of antibiotic resistance in Salmonella." But on the very next page, he states, "Doubtlessly, the majority of resistance in human bacterial populations is due to the therapeutic use of antibiotics in humans."

[9] Ibid., pp. 66 and 67.

human population, so constituting a substantial hazard to human health."[10]

Novick lists sixteen different species of microbial pathogens (including *Staphylococcus, Salmonella,* and *Shigella*) that have been shown to spread from animals to humans. Half of these organisms have also been shown to carry with them antibiotic-resistant plasmids.

Among his more startling conclusions is that the major source of *Salmonella* infections (some 2.5 *million* are recorded annually in the United States alone) is from the contamination of foods *directly* from infected animals. Moreover, he concludes that farm animals contribute between 99 and 99.9 percent of all the resistant coliform bacteria (*E. coli* being the major member) in the environment.

Novick's summary is the most damaging of all. On the basis of his extensive review, he asserts without qualification that the wide prevalence of antibiotic-resistant organisms in the environment is, in his words, "a consequence of massive antibiotic usage in animal husbandry and human medicine." He notes that there are no barriers to the spread of the genes for such resistance, and that they constitute "a substantial hazard to human health due to therapeutic compromise."[11]

Novick thus does not hesitate to state on the basis of his findings that antibiotic feeding is directly responsible for an increase in human disease.

If you were really a skeptic, you might still have challenged these data and their relevance to human health. In fact, if you forced a public health official in 1978 or 1979 to declare that resistant organisms pose a *demonstrable* risk of contagion, someone like Novick might have had to wait to respond. But a clear demonstration of the asked for phenomenon was reported in the February 8, 1980 issue of the *Journal of the American Medical Association.*

[10] Richard P. Novick, "Transmission of Bacterial Pathogens From Animals to Man With Special Reference to Antibiotic Resistance," *Drugs in Livestock Feed,* Vol. II, Background Papers, Office of Technology Assistance, June 1979, p. 3.

[11] Ibid., p. 12.

On August 16, 1976, a routine shipment of calves was made to a dairy farm in northern Connecticut. A not unusual occurrence then went barely noticed: some of the calves showed up sick with diarrhea, and one that had gotten particularly ill in transit died and was buried by the farmer. Four days later, he developed mild diarrhea. Over the next week, the farmer's daughter, though pregnant and near term, nonetheless worked among the calves, scooping milk from a bucket to the calves' mouths with her bare hands as a time-honored way to teach animals to feed from a bucket.

On August 24, the daughter was admitted to a local hospital in labor. The next day she delivered a baby boy. After delivery she had mild diarrhea herself. Three days later her baby showed the same symptoms, and his temperature shot up over 100° F (38° C). Shortly thereafter, two more babies in the same nursery contracted the diarrhea, and in each case, the strain of *Salmonella heidelberg* isolated proved resistant to three different antibiotics (tetracycline, methoxazole, and chloramphenicol).

A detailed epidemiologic investigation revealed that calves from the shipped herds were infected with a strain of *S. heidelberg* which contained the exact same pattern of resistance as the human pathogen. The coincidence of bacterial antibiotic resistance identity and a train of contacts from the farm to the hospital were too stark to be ignored. The authors of the study concluded that they had chanced on the first American demonstration of animal to human spread of a multiply resistant and potentially dangerous strain of bacteria. With characteristic professional understatement, the authors observed that "There has been concern that the use of antibiotics in animal feed might lead to antibiotic resistant organisms or their R-factors could be transferred to human hosts. The present epidemic is consistent with that hypothesis."[12]

Even with the controls instituted under the Swann Committee's report, the situation in Britain deteriorated as well, leading to a critical reassessment in 1979. Citing the epidemics of salmonellosis in the 1960s which originally led to the Committee's appointment, the editors of the prestigious journal *Lancet* decried

[12] R. W. Lyons et al., "An epidemic of resistant *Salmonella* in a nursery," *Journal of the American Medical Association*, 243: 546–47, 1980.

the lack of support for their guidelines and the ineffectiveness of voluntary controls based on prescription practices. Writing in the May 1979 issue, the editors observed that "Ten years after the committee's report, resistant salmonellas in food animals are not even under control, much less eliminated."[13]

Reiterating the theme which by then dozens of researchers had stated, the editors went on to ask, "Is it sensible or even necessary to use chloramphenicol and other agents which can save the lives of human beings, in the treatment of salmonellosis in calves and other food animals? To what extent are antibiotics, prescribed for treatment of infections in animals, being diverted, without veterinary consent, into use to feed animals for promoting growth? Has everyone forgotten the lessons learned in previous outbreaks about the role of bad husbandry in causing infection, and about how good rearing practice can eliminate infection?"

On the basis of such concerns and new evidence brought to light by individual concerned scientists like Novick, congressional circles were stirred to make one more try to restrain the unbridled use of antibiotics in the United States.

CONGRESSIONAL ACTION

In mid-1980, two congressmen, Representatives Henry A. Waxman (Democrat, California) and John Dingell (Democrat, Michigan), had decided to resurrect the FDA's flagging efforts to convince a reluctant public that the future effectiveness of one of their key weapons in the battle against infectious disease was being threatened by the commercial interests of agribusiness. They underscored their position by drafting a bill (H.R. 7285) to restore the power of the FDA to carry out its well-delineated policy to prohibit agricultural enterprises from using major human antibiotics like penicillin and tetracycline to treat their chickens, hogs, and cattle.

[13] Anonymous, "Salmonellosis—An unhappy turn of events," *Lancet*, 1: 1009–10, 1979.

According to an aide, Representative Dingell had decided to push for new legislation in the face of the continuing controversy because he believed the experts were not likely to resolve the issue soon. Dingell himself summarized his position in a letter to *Science* published in September 1980. Noting that the opposition to the restriction on antibiotics is not shared by small diversified producers, who see the reliance on using antibiotics in animal feeds as the primary basis for the growing trend toward large concentrated operations, he observed the following:

> . . . It is this latter factor that goes to the heart of the rhetoric of the Pork Producers and the drug manufacturers—the fear that restrictions on the two most popular antibiotics, penicillin and tetracycline, will stimulate a more critical appraisal of antibiotic use on the part of the entire livestock industry and thereby eliminate the casual consumption and use of these drugs.
>
> It is also common to hear proclamations that the science of this issue is not well understood. There is no question that the therapeutic effectiveness of antibiotics is rapidly diminishing; this decline is directly attributable to the selective pressures of antibiotics. Furthermore, the high degree of similarity of the genes that code for antibiotics resistance from the bacteria of animals and humans leads to the inescapable conclusion that a common selective pressure is at the source of proliferating bacterial resistance. What remains unclear is the precise quantification of the human risk attributable to the use of antibiotics in feeds. However, given that equal quantities of antibiotics are used for therapeutic and feed purposes, the call for quantification will be difficult if not impossible to answer.
>
> The science of this issue is well in hand, but we cannot call upon it to do the impossible. Twenty years of scientific investigation have identified but not quantified the risk to human health. We now face a fork in the road where prudent policy decision and not further study will be the pathfinder.[14]

In fact, the scientific support for this legislation appeared unimpeachable. The same month as the bill was introduced, an article appeared in the *British Medical Journal* which left no doubt of

[14] J. Dingell, "Animal feeds: Effect of antibiotics" (letter), *Science*, 208: 1069, 1980.

the fateful consequences that could attend even the relatively restrictive practices of prescription-based use of antibiotics. Two
years earlier, multiresistant strains of *Salmonella* had appeared in
calves and spread in epidemic proportions through British bovine
herds. In 1979, when animal microbiological records were reviewed, an entirely new strain of *Salmonella typhimurium* was
discovered that proved resistant to seven different antibiotics simultaneously, including the relatively new drug, trimethoprim.

As late as one year earlier, both the pharmaceutical firms that
manufactured the drug and researchers like Dr. H. Richards of
England reported that resistance to trimethoprim was encourag-
ingly rare—less than 0.3 percent of the human *S. typhimurium*
isolated in 1976 and 1977. The drug companies ran ads to this
effect in the veterinary literature.

But in 1979 an outbreak of salmonellosis among calves in at least
50 farms in the South and Southwest of England led to at least
19 human infections and 1 case of fatal septicemia. In all, antibiotic-
resistant *Salmonella* accounted for 310 recorded cases of enteritis—
and 2 deaths in England over a three-year period. All were caused
by strains of *Salmonella* that unequivocally could be traced to animals that had been treated with antibiotics that were otherwise
reserved for treating serious human disease.

In England at least, there was little doubt in 1980 about the consequences of failing to adopt a more stringent policy of controls
than were recommended by the Swann Report. Unfortunately, as
a result of intense lobbying efforts on the part of the pork producers and others heavily invested in retaining complete control
over antibiotic feed supplements, the bill died in committee. Four
years later, researchers at CDC and the Minnesota State Department of Health demonstrated an unequivocal link between an outbreak of salmonellosis in 18 people and *S. newport* from animals
fed antibiotics. The U.S. had its smoking gun.

COST-BENEFIT ISSUES

With a growing reliance on cost-benefit analysis in virtually every
field of regulation, the core issue for reining in antibiotic feed
practices in this country is clearly one of economic relativism.

Even if several hundred cases of salmonellosis were reported here of sufficient gravity to require hospitalization, it is doubtful if the American public would muster the same kind of outrage that greeted the report in the *British Medical Journal* in Britain. The reason is straightforward: The costs of hospitalizing and treating those extra cases of gastroenteritis that might be caused by animal-derived, multiresistant organisms would undoubtedly be shown to be more than outweighed by the economic consequences to agriculture were antibiotics to be curtailed. Agricultural experts allege extraordinary losses would befall the hog or cattle industry were they to be deprived of antibiotic feed supplements, one of the mainstays of efficient production.

Thus, at a cost of $600 a day, and assuming an average hospitalization of 10 days for each of 3,000 salmonellosis patients in this country (proportional to the British statistics), the total cost of roughly $18 million would be dwarfed by the projected loss of "over a half billion dollars" estimated by industry spokesperson Gary L. Cromwell to result if antibiotics were stopped in hogs alone.[15]

What is wrong with such reasoning? For one thing, it counts only the reported cases of salmonellosis, which reflect only about one for every twenty or thirty actual infections. Secondly, it measures productivity and costs to the consumer against the costs—and suffering—borne by those who are involuntary victims of business practices that fly in the face of the recommendations made by governmental agencies. Third, it equates the dollar value of more expensive pork with the short-term costs of hospitalization, without factoring in the possible long-range costs of increased endemic focuses of disease that might also ensue from the policies now in effect. Nor does such an analysis factor in the lost days of productive work—or the human lives lost (estimated to be at least twenty if the outbreak in the United States is anything like that which occurred in England). These last two factors add perhaps another $100 million to the costs.

Even if such an analysis were done, it would be ethically flawed. In the words of the authors of OTA's report on drugs and live-

[15] "Antibiotic Feed Additive Benefits Documented," *National Hog Farmer,* April 1978, pp. 42 and 46.

stock feed, "No common denominator is generally acceptable for comparing human illness and death with pounds of meat."[16]

More critical than the public health implications, however, is the dramatic social dislocation that may result from the unchecked practice of nontherapeutic antibiotic use. The demise of the small farmer and sound animal husbandry; the concentration of wealth in the hands of a few; the profound ecological disturbances that come with mass production; and finally, the dependency of farming enterprises on multinational corporations and the giant drug industries. All of these speak to a broader impact of antibiotic policy.

Could antibiotics be restricted without the staggering costs projected by industry? OTA concluded that the short-term economic consequences could be significant, but costs might be kept down by innovative alternatives. At least one series of experiments suggests that nonantibiotic solutions to calf, and by inference, hog diarrhea caused by *Salmonella* can be readily controlled with a widely available by-product of the feedlots themselves. Researchers at the North Dakota State University Experiment Station have shown that serum taken from mature cattle at slaughter is a ready source of gamma globulin that can protect calves against diarrhea. More importantly, the same "slaughter serum" can be used therapeutically to treat infectious diarrhea that is already under way.

Preventive remedies are of course much more logical, but entail the shift back toward more hygienic practices that often are unobtainable under the economies of scale required by big corporations bent on producing the greatest poundage for the least investment. As we have indicated, antibiotic supplements lose their competitive edge as the conditions of rearing move toward the cleaner and more open patterns of livestock husbandry that were fostered by agricultural extensions in the past.

The trade-off of future assurances of public health safety against the immediate prospects of moderate loss to large cattle and hog farmers might be rectified by approaches already in use.

[16] Office of Technology Assessment, *Drugs in Livestock Feed*, Vol. I: Technical Report, 1979, p. 8.

Government price supports for feed or ancillary support to the farmer, and perhaps even incentives to the pharmaceutical interests to disband their campaign to spread antibiotic use into the stockyard, are one set of options. Direct governmental regulation of the principal nonhuman antibiotics in animal feeds is another.

In the end, it may have to be the farmers themselves who control this dangerous practice, since it is they and their families who are at the greatest risk of contagion and infection with antibiotic-resistant bacteria. Judging from the reports gathered in Missouri, few of the farmers who rely on antibiotics believe that banning them would have a significant adverse effect on their industry. It is only the handful of major users whose incomes exceed $100,000 yearly who declare that restrictions on antibiotic use would hurt them financially. As evidence to the contrary, the Montfort Feedlot operation, largest in the U.S. stopped adding antibiotics to their feedstuffs voluntarily, as did members of the National Cattlemen Association.

Pulling back this marginal aid to mass production would appear to be a small price to pay for the prospect of increased security and reduced risk from the continued spread of one of our nation's most pervasive health hazards.

11

Nonantibiotic Remedies

In an age where everything from colds to acne is treated with antibiotics, it may come as some surprise that some infectious diseases do not need to be treated with antibiotics in order for the patient to recover. Others, like salmonellosis, need only be treated when bacteria invade body tissues. Surprising though reluctant revelations in the medical literature suggest at least three classic cases where antibiotic treatment is unnecessary.

CHOLERA

The first and most dramatic such instance is the dread disease of the tropics—or for that matter, wherever poor sanitation prevails —cholera. Caused by an organism known as *Vibrio cholerae*, cholera has for years been one of the sought after targets of the antimicrobial drug industry. But as with its bacterial counterparts, *E. coli* and staph, the cholera vibrio shows a dramatic and rapid transformation to resistant types when assailed with antimicrobials. Tetracyclines, for instance, can be used effectively *only* if they are given every six hours for two days. Even a slight deviation from this pattern can permit the appearance of antibiotic resistance.

A series of epidemics in Tanzania in the late 1970s illustrates just how dangerous antibiotic dependency can become. By 1978, when a fourth epidemic was under way in almost as many years, the "El Tor" strain of cholera had developed resistance to a multiplicity of antibiotics. As reported by a group of African physician researchers in a 1979 issue of *Lancet,* the vibrio isolated from Tanzanian cases had become resistant to five or six antibiotics in a matter of months after the epidemic began.

By the fall of 1979, the Tanzanian epidemic had spread to Zaire, Burundi, and Rwanda. In Zaire, authorities decided against using the massive application of antibiotics tried in Tanzania, and were able to control the epidemic locally through more traditional forms of cholera treatment: improved sanitation, a reasonably clean water supply, and, for affected children, prompt and effective replacement of body fluids lost from diarrhea. Indeed, rehydration with glucose and balanced salt solutions *alone* is thought by many clinicians to be sufficient treatment for early stages of this otherwise rapidly dehydrating and fatal disease.

These and other experiences have clearly shown that antibiotics are *not* an essential part of effective cholera treatment. But equally important was a lesson learned only with the benefit of hindsight.

In a follow-up report on the Tanzanian epidemic which appeared in *Lancet* on October 20, 1979, four physicians from Belgium made the remarkable discovery that the antibiotic-resistant strains of *El Tor vibrios* imported from Tanzania to Zaire seemed to lose the resistance properties that had been carried on R factors. The most reasonable interpretation for this was the dramatic difference in policy for use of antibiotics in each country: unlike Tanzania, Zaire did not prescribe mass treatments with tetracyclines.

This rapid reversion to an antibiotic-susceptible state has two messages to the medical community: First, it is clear that superfluous antibiotic use can create unnecessary additional risks to the population as a whole by further seeding their microecology with antibiotic-resistant organisms bearing R factors. *Vibrio cholerae* no less than *E. coli* is capable of transferring its resistance genes to other bacteria. (In Tanzania it is highly probable that the now dormant cholera vibrio transferred its R factors to other less visible hosts.) Second, the cessation of unwarranted antibiotic use (as in Zaire) can create conditions that once again permit nonresistant organisms to reemerge and thereby allow a restoration of the status quo whereby the most serious, life-threatening infections can be successfully treated with antibiotics.

The message of the cholera experience is fairly straightforward: Reliance on antibiotic treatment can postpone the development and wide distribution of simpler, more essential therapies. In the case of the initially antibiotic-sensitive organisms, apparent therapeutic success can create a false optimism in having achieved a technological solution for what, in the long run, is essentially an ecological problem involving water quality and personal hygiene.

The medical problem with cholera, as with so many other gastrointestinal infections, is that of restoring the natural flora of the intestinal tract before a child dies of dehydration from diarrhea. A simple solution of glucose or rice with salt has been used successfully to prevent this dehydration and reverse all but the most severe cases of cholera.[1]

TRAVELER'S DIARRHEA

An average of 40–50 percent of all those who travel abroad will discover that one of the hidden perils of their trip is falling victim to the silent epidemic known as traveler's diarrhea. It is less well appreciated that this distressing condition is, in fact, a self-limiting and preventable infection. The condition is both avoidable and responsive to simple remedial treatment.

[1] A. S. M. Mizanur Rahman et al., "Mothers Can Prepare and Use Rice-Salt Oral Rehydration Solution in Rural Bangladesh," *Lancet* ii, 539–540, 1985.

The first reality to appreciate is that traveler's diarrhea is not confined to Mexico. It is a well-kept secret that it is an all too common accompaniment of many of the cruise ships that ply the waters of the Caribbean. (Erstwhile tourists desiring cruise accommodations would be well advised to put in a discreet inquiry regarding the past medical record of the vessel they intend to board since repeat occurrences are the rule not the exception.)

The disease itself is blessedly short lived, but nonetheless brutal in its symptoms. Acute cramping, abdominal pain, and diarrhea are its hallmarks. It is usually caused by a variant of the normal human intestinal bacterium *E. coli,* which has only recently been recognized as having the disturbing ability to produce a toxin. The strain in question is called *enterotoxigenic E. coli,* or ETEC for short.

Apparently, native peoples who have grown up with this type of bacteria have reached a kind of living relationship with them: they are colonized but not victimized. In an ironic twist of history, it is the tourist who is both colonized and victimized. One explanation is that foreigners' *E. coli* have never produced this toxin, and hence the new hosts are physiologically unprepared for the onslaught of this new strain. Like most colonizing species, the ETEC literally take over the intestinal tract, displacing all of the other bacterial types, produce large amounts of toxin that destroy the intestinal lining (pili), and cause massive amounts of fluid to be lost into the intestinal tract.

One of the *worst* means of treating such a diarrheal disease is to prevent the excretion of the toxin in the stools. This is exactly what Lomotil does. It is a drug that prevents the peristaltic movements of the intestines. An equally contraindicated treatment is the use of an antibacterial agent known as Entero-Vioform. Both drugs actually encourage the buildup of the otherwise rapidly dissipated toxin. Entero-Vioform itself can cause severe side effects, which can be fatal. Many physicians believe that the method of choice for treating both ETEC and *Salmonella* diarrheas is symptomatic, using nonopiate pain killers to reduce the discomfort of cramping, and intravenous or oral replacement fluids to restore electrolyte balance.

ETEC is not by any means confined to the tropics. Nor is the

United States exempt from major outbreaks. However, it was not until 1976 that ETEC was shown to cause epidemic diarrhea in American infants. An equally unwelcome surprise was a new and violent epidemic of gastrointestinal disease in Oregon in 1977. At the remote tourist center at Crater Lake, near Eugene, at least 2,310 visitors and 288 staff came down with ETEC diarrhea. Most of the affected persons experienced distress for at least eight days.

In the late 1970s (and even today) it was fashionable for doctors to recommend the use of an antibiotic to treat such traveler's diarrhea. Renowned microbiologists, such as H. L. DuPont of Houston, Texas, whose handbook on antimicrobial use is a classic in the field, may have inadvertently encouraged this practice. In a 1978 paper in the *Journal of Antimicrobial Chemotherapy* DuPont showed that toxin-producing strains of *E. coli* could be typed for antibiotic susceptibility, and by implication, readily treated with an appropriate regimen of antibacterials.

At the same time three British researchers writing in the *Journal of Hygiene* strongly cautioned their peers against using *any* antimicrobial agents to treat traveler's diarrhea. These researchers uncovered the fact that when resistant strains were treated with antibiotics, R factors could be isolated that contained *both* the genes for resistance and those for the toxin, making cross-species spread of pathogenicity an all-too-real possibility. Newly selected strains could become virtual "toxin bombs" for disseminating genes for resistance and toxicity to other bacterial species. Thus, an unexpected side effect of using antibiotics against traveler's diarrhea could be the simultaneous spread of antibiotic resistance *and* enterotoxin production throughout the various bacteria that inhabit the human intestinal tract.

In spite of this most alarming prospect, antibiotics like tetracycline are freely available to "turista" sufferers as an over-the-counter drug in Puerto Rico, Mexico, and other Latin American countries. Most of the available tetracycline ends up being used for precisely this purpose! This, of course, means that resistance will become the rule and not the exception for ETEC.

The development of antibiotic resistance in *E. coli* to the antibiotics marshaled against it could have been anticipated well in advance of the present impasse. As early as 1966, a study of three hundred hospitals in Japan indicated that between 6 and 7 percent of the strains of *E. coli* isolated from the urine of patients with urinary tract infections were capable of resistance to five different antibiotics simultaneously.

By 1971, 8–9 percent of these non-toxin-producing, but nontheless disease-causing, *E. coli* were resistant to six antibiotics. The Japanese epidemiologists cautioned their international compatriots that pathogenic *E. coli* bore the same pattern of resistance on its R factors as did more serious dysentery-producing varieties of *Shigella* and *Salmonella*.

It took almost ten years before an article in a reputable medical journal acknowledged the existence of a simple, time-worn remedy that should make dangerous antibiotic treatments obsolete: bismuth subsalicylate, known more commonly as Pepto-Bismol.

A group of American doctors reporting in an early 1980 issue of the *Journal of the American Medical Association* tested this remedy on a group of U.S. medical students. Because the students were going to spend two or more years in Mexico the researchers reasoned that they would be at a high risk for getting traveler's diarrhea.

The students were divided into control and experimental groups. The object of this carefully designed study was to see if daily use of Pepto-Bismol could reduce their symptoms. The experimental group emerged virtually unscathed, but the doses needed to block the symptoms were rather huge. An accompanying editorial described the amount graphically by advising that travelers who wished to duplicate the test take one or two extra suitcases full of Pepto-Bismol. The editor diplomatically suggesting that the traveler could always use the extra luggage on the return trip for souvenirs. In reality, only small daily amounts of bismuth subsalicylate would likely be needed to prevent traveler's diarrhea.

This relatively simple preparation neutralizes the effects of the toxin, and more significantly, hastens the regeneration of the host's own bacterial population. The more traditional antibiotic regimen of doxycyline at 100 milligrams a day actually *favors* the growth of antibiotic-resistant and toxin-producing *E. coli* strains, increases the risk of the patient's becoming sensitive to sunlight, and encourages the colonization of the intestinal tract with *Salmonella,* a much more hazardous cause of diarrhea. Otherwise it is a perfect treatment!

The message here too is simple. Even the worst cases of infections of the intestinal tract can be self-curing, self-limiting diseases—if you provide an environment that rapidly leads to the recolonization of your intestinal tract with natural flora. Simply choosing treatments that permit this regeneration to occur expeditiously while offsetting the toxic effects of the colonizing bacteria seems to be the method of choice. More to the point, you would probably do best by avoiding the native *E. coli* strains in the first place and sticking with your plan to drink local bottled water or alcoholic beverages.

ACNE

The third and by far most controversial example of questionable antibiotic use lies in the treatment of chronic acne. Anyone who has had to suffer through years of disfiguring facial acne—an experience shared by 30–85 percent of adolescents—knows that acne is by no means a trivial disease. Basically an inflammation of the fat glands at the base of hair follicles, acne has traditionally been treated with drying agents, soaps, and sulfur in various forms.

The acceptance of antibiotics as a justifiable form of treatment for acne has followed a stormy course. In 1969, a "Medical Intelligence" article by Dr. Ruth K. Freinkel in the May 22 issue of the *New England Journal of Medicine* endorsed the use of broad-spectrum antibiotics like tetracyclines as proven and acceptable methods of treatment. Almost ten years later, to the month, an editorial appeared in *Lancet* that decried the use of antibiotics as a "medieval and messy darkness."

The original rationale for antibiotic treatment appeared reasonable enough. Among the antibiotics, only the tetracyclines appeared to interfere with the elaboration of the particular fat-degrading enzyme produced by propionibacteria, which is thought to be linked with these bacteria's acne-producing proclivity.

But in a report of *The Journal of the American Medical Association* on April 25, 1980, three Salt Lake City, Utah, physicians challenged this orthodox remedy. They compared the outcome of sixteen weeks of three forms of therapy, one using large doses of tetracycline and abradant cleansers, a second using the same large doses of tetracycline plus an agent know as tretinoin that reduces the amount of fatty acids in the skin, and a third, using tretinoin along with benzoyl peroxide to minimize skin irritation. Most radically of all, these investigators ordered their teenage patients to *avoid* water in treating their faces, a technique that paradoxically increases the overall moisture content of the skin and thereby changes the microclimate for bacterial growth.

These investigators found that dryness itself aggravated acne, and that their nonantibiotic, topical technique (approach number three above), was as good, or better, than either technique that used antibiotics. Other nonantibiotic agents, like 13-*cis*-retinoic acid, can cure acne, but their use must be tempered by the fact that the drug in question, isoretinoin, can cause birth defects.

These findings, coupled with a growing dissatisfaction among many other clinicians with using tetracycline for protracted periods (up to five years) in treating acne, should provide a welcome alternative to the unnecessary and expensive use of an otherwise valuable antibiotic.

Only time will tell if the medical community heeds the message of these examples: Antibiotics are best seen as the last line of defense against most common bacterial diseases, not the first. In fact, clinicians have only recently accepted that antibiotics have *no* effect on the final resolution of disease processes, even as they are effectively eradicating bacteria.[1]

[1] This controversial position is underscored by L. E. Cluff, "Recovery from infection," in *Clinical Concepts of Infectious Disease,* ed. L. E. Cluff and J. E. Johnson III, 2nd ed. (Williams and Wilkins: Baltimore, 1978); pp. 168–77. Cluff states, "Once injury from infection occurs, elimination of the microbes may prevent further injury; but return to normality is dependent on other events. Antibiotics cannot resolve inflammation, tissue necrosis or pathophysiological processes." (p. 173.)

All of this suggests of course that there is a "better way." What those ways might be are of course currently hotly debated, as moves away from the orthodox methods are met with stiff resistance. Nonetheless, here are a few new approaches.

12

New Approaches to Controlling Bacteria

As a result of reexamination of these and other questionable uses of antibiotics, many physicians and public health officials are being forced to take a closer look at their basic approach to controlling infection. Some believe that reliance on antibiotics has led to a dangerous and pervasive disregard for primary, preventive approaches to control. While our pharmaceutical giants have labored at developing ever more varied versions of chemotherapeutic agents, a few dedicated researchers have chipped away at the core of the problem. Many problems have been posed and resolved.

For instance, what is the source of the pseudomonads that threaten modern-day hospital burn wards? Where are cancer patients getting their exposure to yeasts and fungi that ravage their immunologically vulnerable systems? Why did literally thousands of patients on intravenous fluids develop sepsis? And how can we reduce the risk of infection from catheters?

Some of the answers appear direct and convincing in their simplicity: *Pseudomonas* infection in burn wards can be reduced dramatically simply by screening the diet fed to patients to eliminate foodstuffs shown to be contaminated with *Pseudomonas* organisms. Yeast infections in the cancer ward can be similarly reduced by screening environmental sources of contamination like fruit juices. Contaminated intravenous fluids can be monitored by insisting on prior quality control at the drug companies that make them—and by requiring spot checks in the hospital. Catheter-borne infections can be reduced by adhering to a rigid protocol for changing intravenous tubing, and so on.

It may also be profitable to reexamine the approaches that were proposed by the true visionaries of the microbial revolution. Élie Metchnikoff, Pasteur's contemporary, championed using the innate antagonism between competing groups of microorganisms—some neutral or beneficial, others clearly dangerous—to create an ideal microbial environment.

Since he already had evidence of the protective effect of some bacteria—notably those that accompany extended lactation called lactobacilli—Metchnikoff reasoned that perpetuating the dominance of this flora in the intestinal tract might prove equally beneficial to adults as it appears to be for the newborn. Metchnikoff was singularly impressed with the apparent longevity of Bulgarians who generously laced their diet with yogurt, a good source of lactobacilli.

While we recognize this naïve enthusiasm as amateurish, Metchnikoff's experiments were anything but naïve. He demonstrated that the consumption of systematic doses of acidophilus lactobacteria could transiently increase the content of these beneficial contaminants in the intestinal tract. Indeed, Yale researchers working in a more contemporary setting have shown that two or three 60–90-day periods of daily ingestion of acidophilus-enriched milk followed by 30–50 days without benefit of this diet virtually ensured the permanent colonization of the intestinal tract with these bacteria. Concomitant benefits of reduced intestinal infections could be expected by analogy to the benefits accruing to similarly colonized newborns.

Other avenues of innovation might prove similarly rewarding. Certainly, the dramatic success in recombinant DNA experimentation where the genetic makeup of the experimental and sometimes pathogenic hosts has been altered by inserting new DNA segments suggests an avenue for alternative approaches. Why could not appropriate lactobacilli be genetically programmed to survive and colonize the human intestinal tract, thereby offsetting the risk of gastrointestinal infections of a more dangerous nature? Or why could not recombinant organisms be engineered to synthesize antigenic products to allow for immunization of their hosts?

More to the point, if the *E. coli* that are used in recombinant DNA work have been programmed to lose their ability to receive or transfer R factors—an essential safety step to prevent the inadvertent transfer of genetic material to people—why cannot an R factor be developed that will colonize pathogenic bacteria and "cure" them? Finally, the whole approach of seeding persons with less harmful bacteria to offset possible colonization with more harmful types is an exciting experimental area, albeit one fraught with the ethical problems of human experimentation.

The idea for this innovation can be traced to the work of Louis Pasteur and his colleagues in 1877. Pasteur found that some common bacteria inhibited the ability of virulent anthrax bacilli to cause infections in laboratory animals. In 1909, an opportunity presented itself to test the soundness of this idea in human patients. A man with a severe staph infection of the throat was misdiagnosed as having a case of diphtheria and was sent to the wrong ward. It was common knowledge at the time that patients going to a diphtheria ward who did not already have diphtheria would have it by the time they left. Inexplicably, the staph patient survived.

In a burst of experimental zeal, the attending physician seized on the idea of bacterial competition as the cause of this remarkable case, and sprayed the throats of other diphtheria patients with colonies of the staph carried by his surviving patient. Remarkably (considering the state of hygiene and bacteriology of the time), a significant number of the diphtheria patients recovered!

Over fifty years later, the same idea was tried at a major American hospital. In 1961, a group of newborns at risk of getting a dangerous *Staphylococcus* infection then rampant in the nursery were intentionally seeded shortly after birth with a non-disease-causing staph variety. Called strain 502 A, this nonvirulent staph has been shown repeatedly to provide a remarkable degree of protection to newborns who might otherwise contract a dreaded *Staphylococcus aureus* infection.

While considerable resistance to this idea still persists in the medical community, several hospitals have successfully used strain 502 A to colonize the nose and skin of newborns where staph infections were an imminent hazard. In extended families where chronic infection with other staph strains consistently gave rise to boils and chronic furunculosis, 502 A pretreatment of unaffected family members has also proven remarkably successful in warding off an otherwise likely infection.

Of course, the last point, the relative probability of infection, provides one benchmark against which to measure the ethical acceptability of this approach. If patients are truly at high risk of contracting infection, and if no other means appears at hand to offset it, then experimental therapy with benign colonizers would appear to be a reasonable alternative to offer. Unfortunately, in the past, full disclosure of the possible risks—and the unknown benefits—entailed in this new form of therapy were rarely explored with the patients or their near relatives.

A first principle of antibiosis appears to be fairly well established: Benign strains of various bacteria can provide a protective coating to the skin and mucous membranes that impedes or inhibits colonization with more pathogenic strains. A means of extending this protection could, in theory, be achieved by making the colonizing strains resistant to antibiotics that were to be used systematically to treat infections elsewhere on the person. Researchers ran a test of this theory which utilized the knowledge that certain susceptible patients scheduled to undergo specific forms of surgery would receive a timed pretreatment of massive doses of penicillin. Such treatment would normally wipe out the native strains of bacteria in the throat (*Streptococcus viridians*) and leave the host vulnerable to an overgrowth of more dangerous pathogenic bacteria. (The key to this experiment was the observation that when normal throat bacteria occasionally survived a systemic penicillin treatment no dangerous overgrowth occurred; where they succumbed, it did.)

The researchers therefore reasoned that if they gave a patient just enough penicillin *locally* to select for resistant strains of streptococci in the throat before they gave the massive treatment, the native strains would be protected. Indeed, the results of their trial provided a confirmation of the wisdom of their reasoning: When a group of heart valve patients were given a pretreatment with penicillin intentionally designed to select for resistant strains in the throat, no overgrowth occurred in fifteen out of the sixteen patients. A substantial number of patients in an untreated control group developed the overgrowth with resulting serious infections.

At the end of this study, the authors restated Metchnikoff's fundamental conclusion: Normal bacteria provide a natural host defense mechanism against infection. Unfortunately, even though this experiment constituted dramatic evidence of the ability of intentional selection or seeding with resistant bacteria to protect patients from the overgrowth of harmful bacteria, their findings received little or no attention from the medical community as a whole.

Although numerous disease states, like candidal and trichomonal infections of the vagina, to name only two, are known to be consistently found in patients after antibiotic treatment, little or no attention is yet being given to the approach of controlling the microecology of the patient *before* such treatment to ensure an optimum balance of native host and foreign bacteria.

As a result of investigations such as these, however, our knowledge of the complex ecological relationships among related strains of bacteria has been enhanced. Perhaps more than anything else, this new knowledge has led to a reevaluation of the reasons behind a little understood phenomenon—the gradual appearance of resistance in adults to the strep throat that plagues children.

Detailed laboratory tests on close to a thousand normal persons has recently revealed that on the average each person has a time-dependent increase in the number of indigenous strep bacteria that function as natural bacterial barriers to beta hemolytic streptococcus. As we get older these natural residents acquire the ability to kill the dangerous form of *Streptococcus pyogenes* that causes strep throat.

This study, however, also revealed some disturbing findings regarding antibiotic treatment. In the normal course of streptococcal pharyngitis, or throat infection, the inhibitory microorganisms increase, and remain at this higher level thereafter. But an antibiotic-treated strep throat leaves only weakly inhibiting strep organisms in its wake, making the patient more vulnerable to a secondary infection.

Evidence such as this, while still only suggestive, implies that antibiotics create a kind of closed loop of dependency, first seeming to defeat an infection, while in fact only leaving the host more susceptible for the next bout, thereby creating the need for further antibiotic treatments. These then further impair the survival of the inhibiting microbes that would have made treatment unnecessary in the first place.

With evidence suggesting that this type of pattern is more commonplace than thought previously, investigators are beginning to take bolder, if not more controversial, steps toward new varieties of colonization therapy: seeding susceptible individuals with bacteria able to inhibit more dangerous germs. One example is the intentional seeding of throats of especially susceptible patients with *Streptococcus viridians* (so called because of its ability to turn blood agar green) to offset infection. Another is the use of alpha hemolytic strep to prevent pneumonia in newborns.

Related studies suggest that lactobacilli can protect against gonorrhea by a similar competitive interaction. The evidence is more circumstantial than with the strep story, but still tantalizing. It seems that the two-week period after menstruation, a period during which scientists have recorded the lowest carrier rate for the gonnorrhea organism, coincides with the time when lactobacilli flourish in the vagina. Anecdotal reports of success in using yogurt douches to achieve the same effect are suggestive.

The overall impression from much early research of this kind is that the natural, indigenous microbial flora do indeed confer some protective advantage to each of us. Knowing that we can lose some or all of this protection, even if the loss is seemingly transient, when we are treated with antibiotics should give us pause.

Investigators today liken our natural flora to a protective carpet that is an integral part of our anatomy. Remove the carpet, and you strip away one of the critical layers of our body's defense system, leaving us dramatically more vulnerable to infection.

An approach related to colonization with neutral bacteria has been suggested by microbiologist Debra Jan Bibel. In an unpublished manuscript, Bibel has proposed that bacilli known to produce minute amounts of antibiotics like bacitracin be used to intentionally colonize areas of the skin normally subject to infection with *Streptococcus pyogenes,* the cause of impetigo and pyoderma in addition to scarlet fever and other streptococcal diseases.

According to Dr. Bibel, the administration of microorganisms in the form of replacement therapy is still in its infancy. Its ultimate aim is to provide a period of relative safety by colonizing otherwise susceptible parts of the body in weakened, ill, or aged patients with inhibitory or antibiotic-producing organisms. At least one experiment has in fact been played out with this model in mind. A child whose immune system would otherwise have left it vulnerable to disastrous infections was successfully colonized with a select group of eight different skin bacteria, as well as special bacteria for the throat, nose, and rectum. While this experimental regimen was not entirely successful in affording sustained protection, the whole field of replacement therapy remains an exciting prospect for the enlightened use of bacteria that produce their own antibiotics instead of relying on the broadcast use of commercially manufactured ones.

One simple-minded way to reduce infections is simply to reduce the number of infectious organisms on a given part of the body. Perhaps because of the substantial commercial interest in advancing the claims of the major soap manufacturers, an industry-supported study was done to determine if routine cleansing might make a difference in the incidence of skin infections. The study in question was conducted concurrently at three institutional settings: two at military academies, one in a prison. The pitch in question involved the purported advantages of using deodorants as against plain soaps. The studies clearly showed that routine sudsing reduced the occurrence of serious skin infections, but that the reliance on a deodorant soap conferred little if any real advantage. For instance, over a six-month period of thrice daily washings, only 6 of 599 midshipmen at Annapolis experienced inflamed hair follicles—2 of 602 using the deodorant soap recorded similar complaints—compared to eighteen midshipmen in relatively less-well-cleansed controls.

The key to any real benefit of conscientious soaping appears to hinge on the question of whether or not appreciable reductions of the disease-causing bacteria occur. Here it is well to keep in mind that only 15–20 percent of us actually carry the *aureus* staph on our skin. Soaping reduces their numbers, but only for the relatively dry areas of arms, back, and chest where the organisms are relatively rare to begin with. In the moister areas of the skin (e.g., the armpit, groin, and the webs between the toes) where the organism is usually found, staph withstands the soaping—and actually increases after washing!

As equivocal as washing may be in reducing our own incidence of skin infections, its place in medical practice is not unappreciated. Ever since Joseph Lister showed in 1867 that it was possible to reduce the dreadful 43 percent mortality rate in amputations to 15 percent through the use of carbolic acid and, at about the same time, Ignaz Semmelweis discovered that the terrible scourge of childbed or puerperal fever could be prevented by having medical students wash their hands *before* instead of after birth, surgeons and obstetricians have long recognized that the single most important factor in preventing infection is—not surprisingly—clean hands. Unfortunately, their actions often belie their convictions. A 1981 study of two intensive care unit staffs revealed that physicians (not nurses or medical students) commonly failed to wash their hands between patients.

The bacterial population of the skin is generally made up of two populations, a group of "transients" and the more permanent resident bacteria. When a surgeon washes (or "scrubs" as they term it) he or she first washes the skin with something like a nail brush or some other mechanical scrubber for one or two minutes. This removes dirt, grease, and most of the transient flora. A file is then used under the nails to get rid of accumulated dirt there. Then the actual surgical scrub begins. It is this part of the cleaning process that is directed at the resident flora.

As early as 1938, an observant surgeon named P. B. Price showed that intense washing of the skin brought down the number of bacteria by roughly half for every six minutes of scrubbing. Contemporary thought is that five minutes is about as effective as ten for reducing bacterial counts, and that's about the present limit.

The key to scrubbing (as with much else) is the vigor with which the surgeon brushes the skin. After reducing the germ count to one half or more, a germicidal sollution is used to maintain low bacterial numbers. Chemical agents called iodophors, or more recently chlorhexidine, are active against a broad spectrum of bacteria in keeping the germ counts down after scrubbing. Of course the patient's own skin is also scrubbed the evening before and just before surgery.

The dramatic success of newer degerming methods unfortunately inspired some physicians to institute a disastrous short-cut for controlling staph infections in nurseries. Beginning in Italy, but quickly spreading to the United States and Europe, a degerming agent known as hexachlorophene was used to bathe newborn infants. Like other agents, hexachlorophene left a bacteria-inhibiting film on the skin that allowed progressive washings to build up resistance to superinfection.

But hexachlorophene is heavily contaminated itself—with dangerous dioxins—and exhibits a frighteningly powerful neurotoxic effect. It wasn't until dozens of Italian babies that had literally been dipped into this toxic solution developed paralysis and nerve damage (and some died), that this irrational process was stopped. A final disaster—the explosive dispersion of dioxins from the hexachlorophene factory in Seveso—was the last blow, and hexachlorophene production in Italy was subsequently cut back to postwar levels.

Children in the United States fared better, probably because they weren't immersed in such high concentrations, but the use of hexachlorophene in soaps and over-the-counter medications continued until well after the nerve-damaging effect was publicized and hexachloraphene was made a prescription drug.

The continuing use of hexachlorophene was marred by still another failure, in this case one based on ignorance of the effects of disturbing the complex ecology of microorganisms on the human host. Dr. Harvey Blank, a professor of dermatology at an American hospital, was able to show that the extensive use of this antiseptic permitted the invasion of dangerous *Pseudomonas* bacteria into niches previously occupied by less harmful bacteria.

Today, the simple expedient of hand washing among hospital personnel has come to be recognized as a proven method of reducing the risk of patient infection. In fact, in the words of one clinician, "Hand washing is generally considered the most important single procedure in the prevention of nosocomial infections."[1]

The final conclusion is nonetheless a standoff. Antibacterial soaps are actually the only ones with real inhibiting powers. But they probably belong in the hospital, not in the bathroom. Those bactericidal solutions with appreciable side effects, such as hexachloraphene, are now properly available to the public only by prescription. Deodorant soaps with hyped claims of dramatic inhibiting properties are probably not worth the extra money. Indeed, lack of bathing does not appreciably increase the numbers of skin bacteria in otherwise healthy persons.

Maybe the best solution is, for those of us who can, to get over our preternatural aversions to the germs that find their homes on us. When we are healthy, it appears, so are they.

Time-proven methods of control of infectious disease are thus already making a resurgence. Immunization, as we have already

---

[1] Edward C. Quinn, "Prevention of Bacterial Infection by Non-immunological Measures," in *Current Concepts of Infectious Disease,* ed. E. W. Hook et al. (John Wiley: New York, 1977).

seen in the case of the pneumococcus, is suddenly receiving new attention as a method of controlling newly refractory diseases that only a few years ago were being effectively treated with antibiotics. As knowledge of the basic mechanisms by which bacteria like *Salmonella* and *Shigella* produce their toxic effects, wholly new approaches to developing vaccines have appeared. The very first stages of infection for many of these bacteria has been shown to hinge on their ability to adhere to the surface of the intestinal tract. This adhesion in turn is due to the presence of special bacterial organelles called pili. New vaccines made from these pili alone may well prove to be the answer to preventing widespread infection in susceptible populations.

The most dramatic advances in control of bacterial infection are undoubtedly still to come. Many, such as those involving precisely tailored vaccines or enzyme-resistant antibiotics, will draw from the newly developed recombinant DNA technologies that have permitted the controlled transfer of genetic material from one organism to another. Indeed, the very model on which this technology is based comes from the R-factor story in bacteria. As a deeper understanding of the exact mechanism by which R factors work develops, it will become possible to devise simple genetic variants that can be seeded into bacterial populations that will preclude the transfer of resistance instructions that have so undermined the effectiveness of antibiotics.

With time, a more sophisticated and rational approach will undoubtedly be developed that will allow bacterial infections to be controlled without antibiotics—or where they are absolutely necessary, without the prospect of transfer of those resistance genes that increase the likelihood of broad-scale, uncontrollable infections.

At the core of many of these approaches will be the renaissance of our appreciation of the body's immune system. Already, vaccines to hepatitis B viruses, pseudomonads, and pneumococci have been developed. Others, like a variant of *E. coli* that shares many characteristics of its immune-stimulating antigens with *H. influenzae*, have now been perfected and await clinical trials.

13

Reactivating the Body's Own Natural Defenses

Often lost in the attention given to technological controls to infectious disease is the fact that the body itself is well equipped to deal with most bacterial infections. Indeed, a basic truism of antibiotic treatment is that it just will not work under most circumstances unless the body can mount its own attack against invading bacteria. The body's basic defense system, its immunologic apparatus, augments the action of antibiotics, and if it is weakened, can permit disastrous infections to overwhelm the host. (This is why leukemia patients are so vulnerable to infection even when treated prophylactically with antibiotics.)

The evidence for the critical role of the immune system in the fight against infectious disease comes from the experience of patients whose immune defenses are impaired. In medical language,

such persons are called "compromised" hosts, and for them susceptibility to infection is the rule rather than the exception. Compromised hosts are also liable to unusually severe bouts of disease
once an infection takes hold. Classic examples of such patients
are children with cystic fibrosis, or specific genetically determined
deficiencies in their immune systems, those who lack a spleen, or
have blood diseases like sickle cell anemia or leukemia that indirectly depress the immune system. The elderly and chronic
alcoholics are also typical examples of compromised patients.

For these impaired patients, antibiotic treatment may indeed be
lifesaving, and little or no dispute exists regarding the rationale
for treatment. But understanding just what is missing in the defensive makeup of compromised hosts, has permitted investigators
to augment their therapy and, from animal studies, to piece together a reasonable picture of the normal role of the body's defenses in warding off bacterial invasion and infections.

As early as 1903, two British researchers, P. O. Wright and
A. E. Douglas, discovered that factors in the blood seemed to coat
bacteria and make them much more liable to being taken up by
the body's defensive cells.[1] Today, literally dozens of cells and
chemical factors are known to be involved in a highly coordinated and intricate network of defense that first halts or traps
bacteria, inactivates and neutralizes them, and finally digests them.

The first line of defense is the intact skin and mucous membrane that normally covers all of the body's surfaces. Often, as
we have seen, the bacteria that normally come to inhabit these
surfaces contribute to the resistance of the body to infection with
disease-causing bacteria. Should the skin be broken and bacteria
enter the tissues, they normally encounter an elegantly orches-
trated system of defenses. If the body has previously been infected with the same bacteria and has developed an earlier immune reaction, there is likely to be some antibody present. These
antibodies bind tightly to the molecules that make up part of the
cell wall or capsule of the bacterium. Once attached, they set in

---

[1] Called "opsonins" these serum-borne substances are not recognized as
being essential for the clearance of bacteria, particularly the pneumococci,
from the lungs.

motion a series of other reactions in which small molecules called "complement" bind to the cell wall.

When antibody and complement are both bound to a bacterium, they can cause microscopic leaks in the cell wall, much like those created when a mine is attached to the side of a ship and detonated. In the case of the bacterium, the "explosion" is at a molecular level and is caused by the difference between the internal cellular pressure and that of the outside environment.

In cooperation with other cells, the bacteria are processed and stimulate the production of additional antibody from another population of white blood cells called lymphocytes. Lymphocytes themselves are divided into two groups, B and T, based on the particular organ where they are activated. It is the B type of lymphocyte that makes the types of antibody directed against bacteria. Antibodies, in addition to their direct cell-killing action, can inactivate bacterial toxins or enzymes. When the immune system is particularly vigorous or previously primed by another infection, elimination of invading bacteria can be rapid and virtually total, the whole process taking two to six days.

Antibodies can be of various kinds, each with particular functions and advantages to the host. One type of antibody, called "IgA" (for immunoglobin type A), exerts its favorable effect by coating bacteria in a way that prevents their adherence to body surfaces. IgA antibody is secreted by cells in the intestine and other body lumens. It is also found in tears, milk, and in the secretions of the lining of the air passages.

As you might expect, the bacterial world has engineered defenses here too. Various bacteria have evolved the ability to elaborate enzymes with the specific ability to attack the IgA molecule. Unfortunately, among the most successful antagonists to this very important host defense are the *Neisseria* bacteria that cause meningitis and gonorrhea. (Figures 8 and 9.)

Some complement molecules can also bind, albeit less avidly, to the bacterium's surface even when antibody is absent. Others are designed to attract special white blood cells, known as granulocytes, of which the dominant type is the neutrophil.

A second line of defense is comprised of cells called macrophages that hold invading bacteria in check by literally eating them. This process, called phagocytosis, does not work well against bacteria like the mycobacteria that cause tuberculosis or the salmonellae that cause food poisoning. Both of these bacterial types contain members that can actually thrive in the protected confines of the white cell's interior! Other bacteria, like *Streptococcus pyogenes,* have evolved slippery polysaccharide coats that defy ingestion altogether.

The third line of defense is usually activated several hours after

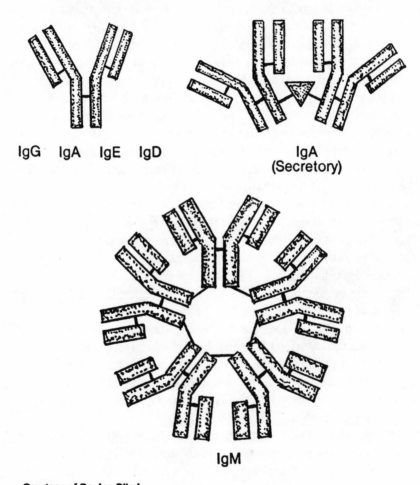

IgG IgA IgE IgD   IgA
                                      (Secretory)

IgM

Figure 8. Immunoglobulins.

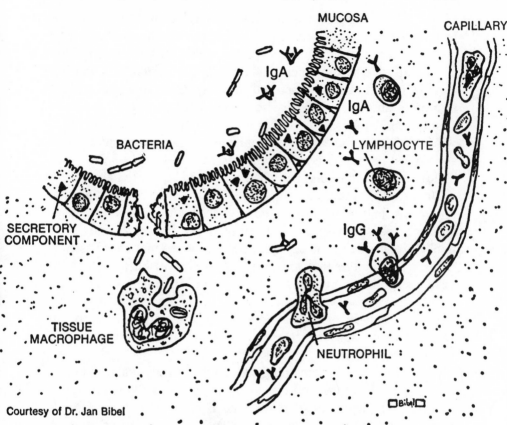

Figure 9. Cellular and humoral defenses.

infection has occurred. It consists of long-lived varieties of macrophages that eat bacteria with great efficiency and specificity and "process" bacterial antigens for presentation to antibody-producing plasma cells.

Obviously, manipulations that improve this front-line defense would appear to offer much promise. Unfortunately, with the notable exception of special derivatives of the pertussis (whooping cough) bacteria and the tubercle bacillus, no sustained effort has been made to devise means of nonspecifically stimulating the body's basic immune defenses. In addition, few physicians have studied the full range of consequences to this primary human defense system posed by the use of antibiotics. Recall that there is almost universal agreement that the effective elimination of an infectious organism requires the cooperation of the patient's own defense system. Most antibiotics, in fact, require the concerted action of all of the components of the immune system to complete their work of thwarting bacterial invaders. Consequently, any action of an antibiotic that adversely affects host resistance could be counterproductive.

In 1977, researchers found that two of the most widely used antibiotics, tetracycline and chloramphenicol, depressed the host's ability to mount an immunologic attack or to scavenge bacteria.

One would think that such a side effect is exactly the kind that physicians cannot afford to ignore in their battle to control dangerous infectious disease. Yet, surprisingly few physicians have publicly expressed concern about the fundamental inconsistency of using antibiotics that are designed to control bacteria, but interfere with the immune system. Many appear to believe that antibiotics can override any impairment of the immune system.

A case study involving patients who are at increased risk of infection because they have lost a spleen provides a testing ground for this proposition.

The spleen works something like an oversized sponge, filtering blood-borne bacterial debris and fostering the activities of many millions of phagocytes. Patients who have lost their spleens, for instance, car accident victims who suffer blunt trauma to their midsections, are, as we have seen, particularly prone to infection. Their susceptibility comes from the loss in both the numbers of defensive cells and the special filtering function. Such patients are particularly vulnerable to getting serious infections caused by pneumococci. For example, as many as 8 percent of splenectomized children experience a life-threatening infection within three years of the loss of their spleens. Most often, the responsible organism is a pneumococcus.

Asplenic patients have thus provided the first testing ground for the concept that antibiotics are indispensable in the treatment of pneumococcal infections. Traditionally, the pneumococci have been among the most sensitive organisms to penicillin, but of late, the problem of resistance to penicillins has forced researchers to look for other means of protecting their patients. Pneumococcal infections resistant to penicillin G occur in up to 5% of patients in some hospitals.[2]

One idea that has surfaced recently is to treat asplenic patients with a vaccine made from the capsules or shells of various types of pneumococci in an effort to stimulate natural immunity in these otherwise impaired hosts. A study begun in England in 1980, headed by Dr. Richard Mayon-White of the Public Health Laboratory Service in Oxford, England, has been started in the hope of thwarting the otherwise highly dangerous pneumococcal infections that afflict asplenic patients. Mayon-White's vaccination protocol promises to reduce the need for maintaining children on penicillin for two to three years, the present preferred treatment.

But the story of the development of the vaccine itself is a disturbing example of a seemingly blatant dismissal of the value of immunologic control measures for treating bacterial diseases.

In the United States, between four and five hundred thousand cases of pneumococcal pneumonia still occur annually—with at least seventeen thousand deaths estimated to occur from what was supposed to have been the disease that penicillin made obsolete. For comparison, note that only about a hundred deaths are charted annually from diseases more commonly linked in the public's mind to health threats (polio, measles, mumps, rubella, diphtheria, pertussis, and tetanus). It is also worth noting that these latter diseases have been brought under control through sustained vaccination campaigns. What is less well known is that effective vaccines for treating pneumonia were tested on American servicemen and elderly patients in the 1940s!

The full story of why this vaccine was effectively shelved for over thirty years remains to be told. Suffice it to say that pneumonia was considered "under control" at various periods during the antibiotic revolution. Where appreciable mortality was common, as among the aged and infirmed, it was euphemistically called by some practitioners, "the old man's friend" in reference to its swift killing effect. In 1974, Theodore Cooper's task force at National Institutes of Health recommended development of a vaccine. It

[2]K. L. Krause et al., "Prevalence of Penicillin-resistant Pneumococci in Houston, Texas," *American Journal of Clinical Pathology* 77, 210–216, 1982.

was not until 1977, however, that the U. S. Public Health Service Advisory Committee on Immunization Practices recommended that a pneumonia vaccine be reinstated into the armamentarium of defenses against this killer. In California, another two years elapsed before legislation was introduced making twenty thousand doses of this vaccine available to high-risk patients, including the elderly who were confined to chronic care institutions.

Why was this action so long in coming? By autumn 1977, it was clear that one of the most susceptible organisms to antibiotic activity, the pneumococci (recall that the first successful uses of penicillin were against pneumococcal pneumonias) was suddenly showing resistance. Over a period of a few months, in South Africa, fifteen children were found who were desperately ill and infected with strains of *Streptococcus pneumoniae* that were resistant to up to five different antibiotics. Two died. That same year, the WHO issued the first of many calls to develop a vaccine to prevent pneumonia in children.

One of the first things that drug companies like Merck Sharp & Dohme of West Point, Pennsylvania, did was to search their arsenals of protective agents for something that would work, particularly in burn wards where patients were increasingly vulnerable to gram-positive infections. MS&D was lucky—in the 1940s they had developed and marketed a vaccine against the surface components ("capsular antigens") of pneumococci, only to find the American medical community less than receptive.

In 1977, they took their vaccine off the shelf, licensed it, and asked for its expanded use. Except for an ill-fated move by the Health and Human Services Administration in 1979 to provide the vaccine to all over-65 Medicare patients, very few physicians have voluntarily chosen to use the vaccine.

Of the developed nations, none had been willing to use the vaccine on the broad scale necessary to offset the threat of widespread dissemination of antibiotic-resistant pneumococci. Only in India were tests of the vaccine begun in earnest—and then only after the encouragement of the World Health Organization.

The strongest voice for developing general immunologic approaches to the increasing threat of antibiotic-resistant bacteria probably belongs to the American physician Dr. William R.

McCabe of the Boston University School of Medicine. Writing in the *Annual Reviews of Medicine* in 1976, McCabe observed that infections with gram-negative, antibiotic-resistant bacteria had reached a rate of 1 percent at some large medical centers. McCabe noted that almost all of the bacterial species represented came from the phylum Enterobacteriacea and shared one or more antigens in common. This fact made vaccination against a spectrum of gram-negative bacteria feasible.

For gram-positive organisms, it may be that physicians will not have a choice in the matter much longer. Total reliance on antibiotics to treat pneumococcal pneumonia may be a thing of the past. In an article appearing in the May 9, 1980 *Journal of the American Medical Association,* researchers report for the first time that high rates of resistance to penicillin of the pneumococci that cause pneumonia are occurring in the general population. Previously, such high relative rates of resistance were uncovered only in confined populations such as those found in the wards of hospitals or homes for the aged.

This article also marked the first time that a broad appeal to consider the use of pneumococcal vaccine was given to the American medical profession. It also is unique in that it includes an injunction to monitor the expected effects of widespread vaccination on the ecology of the pneumococci *before* unanticipated new varieties appear. In this sense, the article breaks new ground and should be given much wider attention than it has received.

Tragically, the Reagan administration has seen fit to delete the funds allocated to Medicare vaccinations, leaving as many as five thousand elderly at risk of dying from pneumococcal pneumonia annually. That numerous patients could benefit from a pneumococcal vaccine in unquestionable, but there are those who, like Albert B. Sabin, developer of the oral polio vaccine, draw the line at giving 25 percent of the population this vaccine. In Sabin's view, "There is . . . no evidence or basis for the recommendation that this vaccine be given to persons over 50 years of age . . ."[3] But

[3] A. B. Sabin, "Immunization: Evaluation of some currently available and prospective vaccines," *Journal of the American Medical Association,* 246: 236–41, 1981.

even Sabin may be wrong. *All* sixty-two elderly pneumonia patients in one study conducted at the Buffalo Veterans Administration Hospital should have received pneumococcal vaccine, according to the physicians who reviewed their charts. Fifty-seven would have been helped by prior immunization. Despite instituting vigorous antibiotic treatment, thirty-two died.

It has become evident that other immunologic approaches could have likewise been developed to treat infections caused by some of the most resistant and pathogenic organisms. A case in point is the use of immunization in the treatment of one of the most common causes of fatal blood poisoning today, anaerobic infections with the bacteria known as *Bacteroides*.

In a 1979 article[4] a group of American researchers dramatically demonstrated the ability of a specially prepared extract of the capsule of this bacterium to prevent otherwise lethal infections. A simple series of injections of the experimental animals with this antigen successfully protected the experimental subjects against challenge with a normally lethal number of *Bacteroides* germs.

The significance of this finding is its date: At least four years before the article appeared, the specific recommendation was made to treat patients (not animals) with such a vaccine, since immunization often provides long-lasting protection for susceptible persons, like the aged, infirm, or immunologically impaired, against such fatal infections of the blood.

Burn patients who might otherwise die from *Pseudomonas* infections are also being experimentally treated by an immunologic approach. At the Medical Research Council's immunology unit in the Birmingham Accident Hospital in England, researchers led by Dr. Roderich Jones, have developed an oral vaccine for burn patients. Unusually fast acting, the vaccine successfully cut mortality in burn patients on whom it was tried by one third. Once successfully immunized, a vaccinated patient's serum can be harvested to treat other patients.

---

[4] J. D. L. Kasper et al., "Protective efficacy of immunization with capsular antigen against experimental infection with *Bacteroides fragilis,*" *Journal of Infectious Diseases*, 140: 724–31, 1979.

What is less evident in this clear triumph is the tension between two competing paradigms of science, immunization, and chemotherapy. In spite of the dramatic success of the New Delhi team headed by Dr. J. L. Gupta in saving eighteen patients in a row with their vaccine, American burn experts, in the words of a January 1978 *Medical World News* article, received the news "almost casually." Among the skeptics was J. Wesley Alexander of the Shriner's Burn Institute, who stated that topical antimicrobials plus sound nutrition work as well or better.[5]

Ironically, the need for such a vaccine was evident years earlier. *Pseudomonas* was becoming increasingly recalcitrant to antibiotic therapy as early as 1971. A general *Pseudomonas* vaccine had even been developed in the early 1970s by Alexander and Bruce G. MacMillan, then Chief of Staff at the Cincinnati Burn Center, but was stopped in 1974. At least four subsequent reports appeared over the next six years demonstrating the efficacy of this procedure for protecting surgical patients against one of the most antibiotic-resistant organisms known. Yet, in 1980, no hospital or major clinic was testing or using *Pseudomonas* vaccine as part of their patient care. In that year, researchers proposed developing a vaccine directed against the toxin produced by *Pseudomonas,* Enterotoxin A, as a highly promising means of offsetting the toxic effects of active infection.

While such vaccines are largely experimental, in the mid-1970s, there was a sufficiently compelling need for further research to have warranted substantially more investments than were actually made. That few embraced this approach as an essential part of preventive medicine or expanded the clinical trials begun in 1968 in Cincinnati on even a scaled down version is alarming.

Another example has been the delay in moving toward non-antibiotic alternatives to protect immunologically compromised

[5] Such a statement runs counter to Alexander's own recommendation four years earlier that "Our results strongly suggest that patients with major thermal injuries should be actively immunized against *Pseudomonas* . . ." J. W. Alexander and M. W. Fisher, "Immunization against *Pseudomonas* in infection after thermal injury," *Journal of Infectious Diseases,* 130: S152–58, 1974.

leukemia victims. For at least twenty years clinicians assumed that leukemia patients are helped by routine treatments with antibiotics to stave off otherwise fatal infections. Actually, in spite of often heroic use of antibiotics, up to 70 percent of leukemia patients commonly die of overwhelming infections. Nonetheless, this questionable practice was not clinically evaluated until the late 1970s. Among the first tests of this otherwise self-evident proposition was one conducted in 1977 by the European Organization for Research on the Treatment of Cancer.[6] In a carefully designed series of experiments on 137 leukemia patients the relative value of ward care, antibiotic treatment, and protective isolation was evaluated.

Three groups of patients were divided among those receiving ward care, protective isolation, and protective isolation plus antibiotics. This last group was given a heavy regimen of antibiotics in addition to their specially prepared hygienic environment. The value of protective isolation became apparent during the course of the study. Significantly more patients on the wards died of infection than did those isolated from unecessary patient or staff contacts.

But adding antibiotics to this protective veil of asepsis added *no* measurable value to the isolation itself. This finding was substantially reinforced by a February 18, 1981 study in the *New England Journal of Medicine* which showed that no additional value was obtained by adding prophylactic antibiotic treatments to the care of acutely ill and immunodepressed leukemia patients.

While *Pseudomonas* vaccine was shown to be effective in reducing the mortality from this common cause of infection in leukemia patients as early as 1974, little follow-up work has been done to apply this promising avenue of therapy over the last seven years.[7]

[6] *Infection,* 5: 107–14, 1977.

[7] Although numerous side effects compromised some of the attempts at immunologic therapy, the leaders of the first clinical trial in 1974 concluded ". . . that reports of decreased mortality due to *Pseudomonas* in certain vaccinated patients makes further study of this preparation advisable." J. E. Pennington, "Preliminary investigations of *Pseudomonas aeruginosa* vaccine in patients with leukemia and cystic fibrosis," *Journal of Infectious Diseases,* 130: S159–62, 1974.

In 1986, little doubt remains that vaccines are invaluable in protecting against some of the most tragic illnesses of childhood and old age. Whooping cough, which caused an estimated 735,000 deaths in the developing world in 1983, is a completely preventable disease. Yet, pertussis vaccine use is declining in part because of exaggerated fears of adverse reaction, an event occurring in only 1 in 310,000 children. Vaccines against ETEC *E. coli* are now possible when they were considered impossible just five years ago.

Pneumococcal pneumonia, which affects up to 570,000 persons in the U.S. annually, is now largely preventable through use of a new, polyvalent vaccine.[8] And acute bronchitis, a major killer among people with chronic lung disease, has recently been shown to be reduced tenfold in incidence by using an easily taken oral preparation of killed *Haemophilus influenzae*.[9] This same vaccine will protect children against otitis media.

Overall, WHO estimates that 15 million children die each year from these preventable causes of acute respiratory infections.

With so much evidence for the failure of antibiotic approaches and such promising successes of immunologic ones, one would think that a wider search for alternatives for treating antibiotic-resistant infections would be well under way by now. That it is not suggests that something is fundamentally wrong with American medicine.

---

[8] See "Update: Pneumococcal Polysaccharide Vaccine Usage—U.S." *Morbidy and Mortality Weekly Report* 33, 273–280, 1984.

[9] R. Clancy et al., "Oral Immunization with Killed *H. influenzae* for Protection Against Acute Bronchitis," *Lancet* ii, 1395–1397, 1985.

14

Conclusion

The period once euphemistically called the Age of the Miracle Drugs is dead. Only the most optimistic observers can believe that we stand much of a chance of recapturing the spirit and hope of that age of some forty years ago. And only the most short-sighted could hope to see a reconstruction of that wonderful era when we believed we were on the verge of chemically conquering all infectious diseases. We tried, and the evolutionary prowess of the microbial world won out.

Many early practitioners believed that the microbial world could be dominated and vanquished by sheer force alone. It is not surprising that some of the earliest clinicians plied their patients with antibiotics in great excess and championed the use of massive intravenous infusions as a means of overcoming any apparent intransigence on the part of the microorganism.

Penicillin, as we have seen, was presented as a wonder drug capable of providing permanent "immunization" against disease. In a popular article written in the early 1940s, a respected scientist heralded it as medicine's "newest and most potent disease destroyer."[1] Glowing tributes like these fostered the erroneous impression that penicillin could be used successfully against *any* infection.

Later, when one antibiotic after another appeared to go into decline, those who stood to gain most by their use advertised gimmicks that purportedly augmented antibiotics' killing power. Antibiotics like streptomycin were prepared as "special salts," or made up in "pH-balanced solution," or injected along with "amplifying agents" that purportedly blocked their excretion from the kidneys—all in the hope of making more dollars on the way to winning the war against the microbe.

When antibiotic use began in earnest in the 1950s, many "new" forms of old antibiotics were produced simply to circumvent medical stagnation or, more often, a patent held by another pharmaceutical company. Irrational use of antibiotics spread, fanned by pharmaceutical house promotions of the invincibility of their new weapons.

Voices of caution were few and far between. A notable exception was Dr. Harris Molliter of the Merck Institute for Therapeutic Research, who in 1946 could already see the problems posed by thoughtless use of penicillin. Speaking at the annual meeting of the Fellows of the American Society of Experimental Biology (FASEB) in that year, Molliter warned that the use of low doses of penicillin in currently faddish products such as lozenges, salves, and tablets invited the emergence of resistant strains. In the face of public statements like this, the argument that antibiotic resistance stemming from the use of these bogus products "took us by surprise" just does not stand up. As we have seen, signs that first sulfa drugs and then penicillin were heading for trouble from resistant strains of bacteria were apparent to many researchers in the very earliest years after their introduction.

Ironically, if we had simply followed the examples of Czecho-

[1] T. E. Stimson, Jr., "Penicillin: New rival of the sulfas," *Science Digest*, 4: 31–33, 1943.

slovakia and Sweden, all that needed to be done to avoid the havoc we have wrought was to hold some antibiotics "in reserve," and call for a moratorium on some others. In this way, the natural selection exerted by continuous application of these potent drugs could have been relaxed, and the natural processes of reversion to the susceptible strains could have ensued. Instead, the American pharmaceutical-medical establishment pursued its chemical attack on the microbial world with a vengeance, and growing numbers of people began to carry the telltale stigmata of excessive antibiotic use: R factors bearing multiple-resistance genes. In turn, the failure of the old drugs stimulated the economics of finding the new, and the treadmill of novel antibiotic production went on and on. This strangely quixotic assault on the microbial world went on unchallenged for forty years.

Such vehement antipathy toward any corner of the living world should have given us pause. Through our related mistakes in the world of higher animals, we should have gained the evolutionary wisdom to predict the outcome.

In Australia we set the stage for a whole continent to be overrun with rabbits because ecologists and naturalists failed to warn against the introduction of a colonizing species into an unoccupied niche. Elsewhere, we have seen entire species annihilated only to be replaced by more dangerous ones as molluscacides, insecticides, rodenticides, and herbicides were used indiscriminately against real and imagined pests. More alarming still, the rapid evolutionary conversion of previously susceptible strains of nematodes, plasmodia, boll weevils, screw worms, caddis flies, mosquitoes, weeds, rats, pigeons, mice, and more, to resistant forms by failed attempts at eradication with similarly toxic chemical poisons provides ample proof of the harmful consequences of blind attempts to subdue the natural world. As the late Robert van den Bosch, champion of integrated pest management, expressed it, "Nature is emitting signals saying that we cannot continue our attempts to ruthlessly dominate her and that if we persist, disaster is in the offing . . ."[2]

Underestimating the evolutionary potential of living organisms

---

[2] Robert van den Bosch, *The Pesticide Conspiracy* (Doubleday: New York, 1978).

is the single most important mistake made by those who use chemical means to subdue nature. The ability to withstand human onslaught and rebound seemingly twice as strong as before is a common theme that pervades the mythology of many cultures. Greek legend has it that only Hercules could successfully outfight Hydra, the snake-headed monster who would grow back two heads for every one cut off. The derivative myth of Medusa confronts rational man with the paradox we have been exploring: How can human invention cope with radical change without the kind of paralysis that grips most of us in the face of a totally alien transformation of nature?

Such blindness toward evolutionary change is at one and the same time the cause for much of the present dilemma of therapeutic ineffectiveness against bacteria, and the source of continued concern for the ensuing consequences of such neglect. Without this evolutionary perspective, we are not only likely to continue to lose the war against the microbes, but we may very well push ourselves into an evolutionary end game with our bacterial parasites and commensals in which even our most ambitious and imaginative approaches for control are doomed to fail.

Similar arguments must now be mustered against the medical establishment. Our preference for chemical assaults over immunological approaches reveals a cultural bias that values treatment over prevention. We favor simple technological fixes for complex disease entities, while our medical complex fosters a near-sighted one-germ, one-chemical mentality. Together, these positions contribute to a world view that encourages the proliferation of new chemotherapeutic agents, and in turn, the proliferation of new disease entities.

The cultural reinforcement for a reliance on antibiotics is revealed not only in their prevalence as prescription drugs (second only to tranquilizers), but to their continued proliferation in spite of a growing litany of treatment failures. Only about one in every thousand antibiotics ever gets marketed, and the success rate is plummeting as the competition from bacteria more resistant than their predecessors gets stiffer. Add to this dilemma the finite possibilities of synthesizing new chemical structures for antibiotics that can "beat the resistance game," and you have a dismal picture indeed.

The losers in this race, however, are unlikely to be the pharmaceutical giants, who, like Lilly and Pfizer, have maintained their supremacy in marketing antibiotics for over three decades. The real losers are more likely to be the patients and the public who are tended by chemical-minded, conservative clinicians.

We are at a time in the history of control of infectious disease when the public may greet each new chemotherapeutic discovery, in the words of playwright Bertolt Brecht, "with howls of despair." Where are the champions of naturopathic medicine? Where are the Metchnikoffs of our time? Why must we endure this economic pestilence of chemicals-for-profit when public health approaches go wanting?

Where are those who believed that most infectious diseases are generated by ecological imbalances? Where are those who have supplanted the wish to dominate the microbial world with the conviction that seeking an integrated approach to control is in the end the only way out?

Using chemicals that are derived from substances used in nature to control bacteria—or insect pests—is in itself a reasonable approach. Such antibiotics, or their pesticide equivalents in pyrethrins, are probably intrinsically safer and less toxic than most synthetic analogs that depend on adding reactive groups that have not been subjected to the kind of evolutionary scrutiny that characterizes the "natural" toxins.

But the very origins of these means should have alerted scientists to the pitfall in the end: If such substances occur widely in nature, natural systems will have devised means to bring them into balance. Where technological intervention goes awry, it is often because such natural balancing forces were ignored. In each case, someone, somewhere failed to recognize a key biological attribute of the organisms being attacked. And for the organisms that concern us here, the single most important attribute ignored has been their ability to undergo genetic change and adaptation, and via R factors, to disperse this ability throughout the microbial world.

The lesson from both our agricultural and medical experience is remarkable for its consistency: Ignoring the evolutionary attributes of biological systems can only be done at the peril of ecological catastrophe.

The reasons for such a gloomy prospect are clear: economic incentive to develop ever more refined and novel products, medical unwillingness to accept the guidance of peer review committees at hospitals, stubborn and often blind commitment to a substance that "always worked in the past," and the presumptuousness that says that chemical control over an evolutionarily subordinate organism is always more desirable than biological control.

These factors together with a blind belief in the "magic bullet" approach of medicine create a philosophical orientation to control of infection that places more and more Americans at the hands of practitioners with an evolutionary and therapeutic blind spot. Those who control the access to prescription drugs can unwittingly wall off opportunities for meaningful approaches in self-help and genuine advances in immunology that would have the body's own defenses control infection.

The answer clearly does not consist of throwing more troops into a losing battle. Simply adding new variations onto old antibiotic themes has not worked. And every year snowing the medical community with a host of "new" antibiotics that merely compound the community problems of control has not proven to be the answer either.

Even the most successful of the new combination antibiotics like trimethoprim-sulfamethoxazole leave much to be desired as effective means of offsetting the constant epidemiologic problem of novel genetic combinations in newly emergent strains. Even this most widely heralded "wonder drug" has failed to control some forms of infection—and its overuse has led to the selection of still a third generation of resistant organisms.

What is remarkable about all this is not so much that enormous amounts of chemical inhibitors, toxins, or otherwise lethal agents have been directed at a single phylum (no one questions the relative undesirability of human pathogens compared, say, to that of the sea otter), but rather that this wholesale onslaught has been undertaken without the slightest concern for its vast evolutionary consequences, and has resulted in often very damaging biological imbalances.

At least three factors have led to this dreadful outcome. The first was the medical profession's inability to recognize the complex interactions that link bacterial species and to incorporate that knowledge into rational medical practice. The failure to recognize basic principles of infection control and medical epidemiology can be traced to the fact that American physicians receive substantially less training in microbiology and bacteriology (as well as the related specialty of immunology) than do their European counterparts.

Microbiology, the customary showplace for theoreticians of the old schools of bacteriology and immunology, has become an elective course at all but the most traditional American medical schools. At many institutions, the falloff from 1968 to 1978 in the number of hours devoted to the study of microbiology plummeted by half. According to experts in medical education, some school faculties have come to operate as if infectious diseases are somehow entities of a bygone era.

Choice and judicious use of carefully defined antibiotics to counter diseases that the hospital or outside testing service has diagnosed for the physician have become the mainstay of instruction at most medical schools. As a result, many new interns emerge unaware, in the view of Dr. Calvin Kunin, of even the basic concepts of infection control. In such a climate of ignorance, is it any wonder that many physicians apply antibiotics by rote, and turn to the often misleading circulars of the pharmaceutical manufacturers for guidance?

The ignorance displayed by the proponents of broad-spectrum antibiotics is analogous to the mind-set of the advocates of broad-spectrum pesticides like DDT, or dioxin-contaminated toxaphene or pentachlorophenol, who failed to recognize the long-term consequences of using such potent, long-lived poisons. All of these agents not only generated resistance among the organisms that they were used to treat, but also have caused major perturbations in the ecosystems in which they were used.

By ignoring the delicate balance that characterizes the web of

life among the organisms in the microbial world, wanton antibiotic use caused similar disturbances, disturbances whose full
ramifications are just now beginning to be understood.

Both groups of nonspecific toxins produced the same predictable outcome: the overgrowth of resistant or novel organisms and
unanticipated outbreaks of new diseases or pestilence.

The second factor contributing to the demise of the usefulness
of antibiotics was the entrepreneurial bent of the pharmaceutical
manufacturers among the hundred and forty or so companies in
the United States whose drive to put competitive products on
the market often ran roughshod over normal controls on quality
or safety—and more ominously on the rational practice of
medicine. Letting marketplace considerations outstrip the public
weal is a common problem among the so-called ethical pharmaceutical purveyors. What was new with antibiotics was the
almost total disregard of medical advice among many of their
most knowledgeable experts. The documentation of the history of
this pattern is laid out in the book by Silverman and Lee mentioned in Chapter 1, *Pills, Profits and Politics*.

The third and most disturbing factor has been the preoccupation of physicians themselves with patient needs over the more
global needs of the public. Catering to patient requests in the
prescription of antibiotics is a well-known problem among private
and hospital physicians. Even in the face of the emergence of resistant strains, many physicians continue to prescribe antibiotics
that are either contraindicated or unlikely to be effective at the
dosages employed.

It is as if the promise of a quick fix to livestock management or
to a patient's immediate health needs is more important than the
more long-term needs for community safety that would require
careful development of a rational policy for the use of antibiotics.
This preoccupation with a chemical solution to infectious disease
has set back valuable immunological and other nonchemical
approaches years. The development and marketing of vaccines
like that for pneumococcal pneumonia or *Pseudomonas* were
delayed or even shelved after initial successful development in
preference to an antibiotic solution. Now that the solution is no
longer working, these same vaccines should be reactivated and

made widely available. That they are not (witness the cancellation of Medicare payments for pneumococcal vaccine), is a national disgrace.

So what should have been perceived as a complex problem that required collective solutions must now be taken from the hands of individual practitioners. We can no longer stand frozen in the face of these new circumstances.

To this day we still tolerate the uncontrolled and virtually unregulated use of antibiotics in animal feeds as well as in hospitals, in spite of recommendations from our own commissions and those of the British. Both our own Food and Drug Administration panels and the august Swann Committee have urged more rational policies. But the demand for continued individual discretion and *laissez-faire* economics threatens to hold any successful implementation of these recommendations in abeyance.

Instead of the firm rules governing antibiotic use that have been developed in public-health-conscious countries like Sweden, Czechoslovakia, and Japan, the United States has adopted "voluntary" hospital surveillance programs or "guidelines" for the rational use of antibiotics in general hospitals. Private practice and surgical suites have proven virtually immune from outside interference.

As long as quasisolutions like these are in effect, the continued proliferation of new antibiotics and the uncontrolled use of those already on the market is guaranteed.

What then is the answer to the dilemmas posed by this phenomenon? The step that should be taken immediately as a national priority, is to designate some antibiotics for emergency use only. This could be readily achieved by limiting those key antibiotics to hospital use only, and designating the local Infection Committee or like unit, as the arbiter of when they were to be used. Holding some antibiotics in reserve has been an established practice in countries like Sweden for many years. The rationale behind this policy is straightforward. By keeping certain antibiotics out of mainstream practice, you ensure that when they are used, most of the target organisms will be sensitive to their inhibiting or killing effect. While this policy does not always work —for instance, if other hospitals in the same area follow divergent strategies—its successful application has already been demonstrated in the United States.[8]

The second step is to restrict all nontherapeutic uses of antibiotics in animal feeds, and to limit their uses in therapy to a group of antibiotics that differs from those used to treat human infections. The rationale here is again straightforward: even where nonhuman antibiotics are used in animal feed, the risk remains that selection for R-factor-bearing bacteria will still occur—and that cross-resistance to antibiotics intended for human use may happen as it does in the case of chloramphenicol.

The third step is to restrict antibiotic use in office practice by increasing the surveillance of peer review committees and alerting physicians to the prospects of wider dissemination of antibiotic-resistant strains within their own communities. Better patient education, through the reactivation of the notion of providing patient-directed package inserts, would also reduce the expectation of antibiotic prescriptions for nonessential infections.

The fourth step is to clamp down further on the already recognized misuses of antibiotics in hospital settings through the reinforcement of existing review procedures, audits, and censure processes already in place. Hospital administrators need to recognize the gravity of continued neglect, and the consequences, monetary and health, that ensue from neglect of rigorous control over antibiotic use.

At an international level, firm peer pressure to bring all prescription practices into line with rational medicine is obviously critical.

In the end it is crucial to recognize that the strengths of human invention in coping with the antibiotic morass most definitely do

[8] At the University of Florida's Shands Teaching Hospital in 1970, 96 percent of the staphylococcus strains tested proved sensitive to erythromycin, a dramatic contrast to the high rates of resistance found elsewhere in the country. The reason for this turnabout proved to be the conscious policy to restrict prescriptions for erythromycin—only two prescriptions had been written in the previous three years. Similar success has been recorded elsewhere with antibiotic-resistant *Klebsiella*, where an outbreak of infection was halted by prohibiting the practice of routinely using ampicillin and cloxacillin.

not include the kind of synthetic approach needed to cope with a problem as multifarious, even global, as is that of antibiotic resistance. Thus, while we can and have used the most sophisticated technology to classify and identify microorganisms, to synthesize extraordinarily complex biochemical molecules, and to measure precisely the number and kind of individual bacteria in a complex mixture from a human patient, we have failed to appreciate the evolutionary basis for the emergence of antibiotic resistance or the complex arguments in favor of vaccines. Nor have we understood their interrelationships or predicted accurately the global outcomes of our interventions. Indeed, the emergence of antibiotic resistance and its uncontrolled spread stands as a stark reminder of the narrowness of our collective medical wisdom and our unwillingness to put the public good over that of the individual.

15

Epilogue: The Medusa Effect Revisited

The demise of Medusa in the hands of Perseus carries a final message. With Medusa's death, Perseus received two drops of her blood to give to the goddess Athena. One drop had the power to kill and spread evil through the world, the other, to heal and restore well-being. Athena in her wisdom conveyed the second drop to Asclepius, considered the founder of Western medicine.

As we painfully take stock of our hubris in assuming that we can control the transformations of nature, we might ponder the choices open to us. We can either use our control over the bacterial world to spread an incomplete cure to what is certainly a worldwide problem of antibiotic resistance, or we can look toward the new methods for controlling and living with the microbial world. If Asclepius' charge means anything, it is that we can

no longer afford to treat problems of this magnitude in isolation
from the world community.

Nothing short of a collective agreement to use antibiotics according to recognized international policies of public health will
suffice to restore the Asclepian authority so sorely lacking in the
area of microbial medicine.

Bibliography

CHAPTER 1   INTRODUCTION: THE MEDUSA EFFECT

Anderson, E. S. "Drug resistance in Salmonella typhimurium and its implications," *British Medical Journal*, 3: 333–39, 1968.

———. "Middlesbrough outbreak of infantile enteritis and transferable drug resistance," *British Medical Journal*, 1: 293–95, 1968.

Anonymous. "Antibiotic audit," *Lancet*, 1: 310–11, 1981.

Anonymous. "Hospital germs eyed," *Modern Healthcare*, March 1979, p. 21.

Anonymous. "Infections due to penicillinase-producing *Neisseria gonorrhea*—Florida," *Morbidity and Mortality Weekly Report*, 30: 245–47, 1981.

Anonymous. "Multiply resistant pneumococcus—Colorado," *Morbidity and Mortality Weekly Report*, 30: 197–98, 1981.

Anonymous. "Resistance to antibiotics," *Journal of the American Medical Association*, 203: 1132, 1968.

Bartlett, J. G., et al. "Cephalosporin-associated pseudomembranous colitis due to Clostridium difficile," *Journal of the American Medical Association*, 242: 2683–85, 1979.

Falkow, S. "Antibiotic resistance of gram-negative microorganisms," *Medicus,* University of Washington, Winter, 1976, pp. 3–9.

Florey, Sir Howard. *Antibiotics.* Alden & Blackwell: Windsor, England, 1951.

Galdston, I., ed. *The Impact of Antibiotics on Medicine and Society.* New York Academy of Medicine: New York, 1958.

Gardner, P. "When is antibiotic therapy appropriate?" *Drug Update,* January 1977, pp. 31–36.

Jacobs, M. R., et al. "Emergence of multiply resistant pneumococci," *New England Journal of Medicine,* 299: 735–40, 1978.

Kunter, E. "Sensitivity of mastitis pathogens to antibiotics and chemotherapeutic agents," *Archives of Experimental Veterinary Medicine,* 29: 1–32, 1975.

Kuwahara, S., et al. "Transmission of multiple drug resistance from Shigella flexneri to Vibrio comma through conjugation," *Japanese Journal of Microbiology,* 7: 61–68, 1963.

Martys, C. R. "Adverse reactions to drugs in general practice," *British Medical Journal,* 2: 1194–97, 1979.

Platt, D. J. "Prevalence of multiple antibiotic resistance in *Neisseria gonorrhoeae,*" *British Journal of Venereal Disease,* 52: 384–86, 1976.

Powell, R. D., and Tigertt, W. D. "Drug resistance of parasites causing human malaria," *Annual Review of Medicine,* 19: 81–102, 1968.

Remington, J. S. "Trouble with antibiotics," *Human Nature,* June 1978, pp. 62–71.

Rowe, B., et al. "Epidemic spread of *Salmonella hadar* in England and Wales," *British Medical Journal,* 1: 1065–68, 1980.

Ryder, R. W., et al. "Infantile diarrhea produced by heat-stable enterotoxigenic *Escherichia coli,*" *New England Journal of Medicine,* 295: 849–53, 1976.

Shtibel, R. "Resistance of Neisseria gonorrhoeae to antibacterial drugs in Ontario," *Health and Laboratory Science,* 13: 49–53, 1976.

Silverman, M., and Lee, P. R. *Pills, Profits and Politics.* University of California Press: Berkeley, 1974.

Sparling, P. F., et al. "Inheritance of low-level resistance to penicillin, tetracycline and chloramphenicol in *Neisseria gonorrhoeae,*" *Journal of Bacteriology,* 124: 740–49, 1975.

Sugarman, B., and Pesanti, E. "Treatment failures secondary to in vivo development of drug resistance by microorganisms," *Reviews of Infectious Diseases,* 2: 153–68, 1980.

Threlfall, E. J., et al. "Plasmid encoded trimethoprim resistance in multiresistant epidemic *Salmonella typhimurium* phage types 204 and 193 in Britain," *British Medical Journal,* 1: 1210–12, 1980.

Watanabe, T. "Infectious drug resistance," *Scientific American,* 217: 19–27, 1967.

Welch, H. "Antibiotics 1943–1955: Their development and role in present-day society," in Galdston, pp. 70ff.

CHAPTER 2   THE EXTENT OF THE PROBLEM

Andriole, V. T. *"Pseudomonas* bacteremia: can antibiotic therapy improve survival?" *Journal of Laboratory and Clinical Medicine,* 94: 196–200, 1979.

Atkinson, B., and Moore, G. "A sample of bacterial isolates in the United States and their susceptibilities to antimicrobial agents," in *Significance of Medical Microbiology in the Care of Patients,* ed. V. Lorian. Williams & Wilkins Co.: Baltimore, 1976.

Baker, C. J., and Barrett, F. F. "Group B streptococcal infections in infants; the importance of the various serotypes," *Journal of the American Medical Association,* 230: 1158–60, 1974.

Baldwin, R. A. "Development of transferable drug resistance in *Salmonella* and its public health implications," *Journal of the American Medical Association,* 157: 1841–53, 1970.

Bruun, J. N., et al. "Epidemiology of *Pseudomonas aeruginosa* infections: Determination by pyocin typing," *Journal of Clinical Microbiology,* 3: 264–71, 1976.

Cherubin, C., et al. "Recent trends in salmonella and shigella at Kings County Hospital," *Bulletin of the New York Academy of Medicine,* 55: 303–12, 1979.

Cooper, T. "Infectious disease: No cause for complacency," *Journal of Infectious Diseases,* 134: 510–12, 1976.

Dixon, R. E. "Effect of infections on hospital care," *Annals of Internal Medicine,* 89 (Part 2): 749–53, 1978.

————. "Epidemiology of drug resistance in hospitals," in *Drug-Inactivating Enzymes and Antibiotic Resistance,* ed. S. Misuhashi et al. Springer-Verlag: New York, 1975; pp. 349–60.

Driessen, J. H. "A computerized study of bacterial resistance patterns (1971–1974)," *Scandinavian Journal of Infectious Disease (Supplement),* 9: 67–71, 1976.

Dubos, R. *Mirage of Health: Utopias, Progress and Biological Change.* Doubleday: Garden City, N.Y., 1959.

Echeverria, P., et al. "Antimicrobial resistance and enterotoxin production among isolates of Escherichia coli in the Far East," *Lancet,* 2: 589–92, 1978.

Finkel, M. J. "Magnitude of antibiotic use," *Annals of Internal Medicine,* 89 (Part 2): 791–92, 1978.

Finland, M. "And the walls come tumbling down: more antibiotic resistance, and now the pneumococcus," *New England Journal of Medicine,* 299: 770–71, 1978.

————. "Changing patterns of common bacterial pathogens to antimicrobial agents," *Annals of Internal Medicine,* 76: 1009–13, 1972.

————. "Superinfections in the antibiotic era," *Postgraduate Medicine,* 54: 175–83, 1973.

Freeman, J., et al. "Adverse effects of nosocomial infection," *Journal of Infectious Diseases,* 140: 732–40, 1979.

Galbraith, N. S., et al. "Changing patterns of communicable disease in England and Wales," *British Medical Journal,* 281: 427–30; 489–92; 546–49, 1980.

Hansman, D. "Haemophilus influenzae type B resistant to tetracycline isolated from children with meningitis," *Lancet,* 2: 893–96, 1975.

Jacobs, M. R., et al. "Emergence of multiply resistant pneumococci," *New England Journal of Medicine,* 299: 735–40, 1978.

Kobari, K., et al. "Antibiotic-resistant strains of El Tor vibrio in the Philippines and the use of furalazine for chemotherapy," *Bulletin of the World Health Organization,* 43: 365–71, 1970.

Kunin, C. M. "Antibiotic accountability," *New England Journal of Medicine,* 301: 380–81, 1979.

———., et al. "Use of antibiotics: A brief exposition of the problem and some tentative solutions," *Annals of Internal Medicine,* 79: 555–61, 1973.

Kwitko, A. O., et al. "Serratia: opportunistic pathogen of increasing clinical importance," *Medical Journal of Australia,* 2: 119–21, 1977.

McCabe, W. R. "Immunoprophylaxis of Gram-negative bacillary infections," *Annual Reviews of Medicine,* 72: 335–41, 1976.

McKeown, T. "A historical appraisal of the medical task," in *Medical History and Medical Care: A Symposium of Perspectives,* ed. T. McKeown and G. McLachlan. Oxford University Press: New York, 1971; pp. 29–55.

———. *The Modern Price of Population.* Academic Press: New York, 1976.

Millar, J. W., et al. "In vivo and in vitro resistance to sulfadiazine in strains of *Neisseria meningitidis,*" *Journal of the American Medical Association,* 186: 139–41, 1963.

Moffet, H. L. "Common infections in ambulatory patients," *Annals of Internal Medicine,* 89 (Part 2): 743–45, 1978.

Mufson, M. A., et al. "Capsular types and outcome of bacterial pneumococcal diseases in the antibiotic era," *Archives of Internal Medicine,* 134: 505–10, 1974.

National Center for Health Statistics, Births, Marriages, Divorces and Deaths for March 1981, Vol. 30(3), June 11, 1981.

National Center for Health Statistics Monthly Vital Statistics Report: Provisional statistics annual summary for the United States 1978, Vol. 27, No. 13. Rockville, Md.: National Center for Health Statistics, 1979; Table 10 (DHEW Publication Number PHS79-1120).

Platt, D. J. "Prevalence of multiple antibiotic resistance in *Neisseria gonorrhoeae*," *British Journal of Venereal Disease*, 52: 384–86, 1976.

Pollock, A. V., and Evans, M. "Changing patterns of bacterial resistance to prophylactic use of cephaloridine and therapeutic use of ampicillin," *Lancet*, 2: 1251–54, 1975.

Renaud, M. "On the structural constraints to state intervention in health," in *Health and Medical Care in the U.S. A Critical Analysis*, ed. V. Navarro. Baywood Publishing Co.: Farmingdale, N.Y., 1975; pp. 135–46.

Richmond, A., et al. "R-factors in gentamicin resistant organisms causing hospital infection," *Lancet*, 2: 1176–78, 1975.

Robinson, R. A. "Antibiotic resistance of shigellas in New Zealand," *New Zealand Medical Journal*, 83: 81–82, 1976.

Salzman, T. C., et al. "Shigella with transferable drug resistance: outbreak in a nursery for premature infants," *Journal of Pediatrics*, 71: 21–28, 1967.

Scheckler, W. E., and Bennett, J. V. "Antibiotic usage in seven community hospitals," *Journal of the American Medical Association*, 213: 264–70, 1970.

Siebert, W. T., et al. "Resistance to gentamicin: A growing concern," *Southern Medical Journal*, 70: 289–92, 1977.

Siegal, J. D., et al. "Single dose penicillin prophylaxis against neonatal Group B Streptococcal infections," *New England Journal of Medicine*, 303: 769–75, 1980.

Simmons, H. E., and Stolley, P. D. "This is medical progress? Trends and consequences of antibiotic use in the United States,"

Journal of the American Medical Association, 227: 1023–28, 1974.

Smith, D. H. "Salmonella with transferable drug resistance," *New England Journal of Medicine,* 275: 625–28, 1966.

Stollerman, G. H. "Trends in bacterial virulence and antibiotic susceptibility: Streptococci, pneumococci and gonococci," *Annals of Internal Medicine,* 89 (Part 2): 746–48, 1978.

Wynne, J. W. "Pulmonary disease in the elderly," in *Clinical Geriatrics,* 2nd ed., ed. I. Rossman. J. B. Lippincott Company: Philadelphia, 1979; pp. 239–65.

CHAPTER 3   THE QUEST FOR MIRACLE DRUGS

Abraham, E. P. "The beta-lactam antibiotics," *Scientific American,* 244: 76–87, June 1981.

————, and Chain, E. "An enzyme from bacteria able to destroy penicillin," *Nature,* 146: 837, 1940.

Anonymous, *Profile of An Antibiotic, Keflin Sodium Cephalothin.* Eli Lilly & Co.: Indianapolis, 1966.

Florey, H. W. "Clinical uses of penicillin," *British Medical Bulletin,* 2:9–13, 1944.

Garrod, L. P. "Penicillin: its properties and powers as a therapeutic agent," *British Medical Bulletin,* 2: 2–7, 1944.

Lacey, R. W., and Lord, V. L. "New type of β lactam resistance in *Staphylococcus aureus,*" *Lancet,* 1: 1049–50, 1981.

Macfarlane, G. *Howard Florey.* Oxford University Press: London, 1979.

Marti-Ibanez, F. *Men, Molds, and History.* MD Publications, Inc.: New York, 1958.

McKee, C. M., and Houck, C. L. "Induced resistance to penicillin of cultures of staphylococci, pneumococci and streptococci," *Proceedings of the Society for Experimental Biology (New York),* 53: 33–38, 1943.

Ory, E. M., et al. "Bacteriologic studies of the sputum of patients with pneumococcic pneumonia treated with penicillin," *Journal of Laboratory and Clinical Medicine,* 31: 409–13, 1946.

Schmidt, L. H., and Sesler, C. L. "Development of resistance to penicillin by pneumococci," *Proceedings of the Society for Experimental Biology (New York),* 52: 353–60, 1943.

Strome, M. "Unresponsive acute otitis media: Comments," *Pediatric Alert,* 6: 42, May 28, 1981.

CHAPTER 4   HOW DO ANTIBIOTICS WORK?

Acar, J. F., and Sabath, L. D. "Bacterial persistence in vivo: resistance or tolerance to antibiotics," *Scandinavian Journal of Infectious Disease (Supplement),* 14: 86–91, 1978.

Anonymous. "The clinical significance of tolerance of Staphylococcus aureus," *Annals of Internal Medicine,* 93: 924–26, 1980.

Barry, A. L. *The Antimicrobic Susceptibility Test: Principles and Practices.* Lea and Febiger: Philadelphia, 1976.

DuPont, H. L. *Practical Antimicrobial Therapy.* Appleton-Century-Crofts: New York, 1978.

Eichenwald, H., and McCracken, Jr., G. H. "Antimicrobial therapy in infants and children," *Journal of Pediatrics,* 93: 337–77, 1978.

Eickhoff, T. C., and Finland, M. "Changing susceptibility of meningococci to antimicrobial agents," *New England Journal of Medicine,* 272: 395–98, 1965.

Geddes, A. M. "Use of antibiotics: septicaemia," *British Medical Journal,* 2: 181–84, 1978.

Levison, M. E. "Antibiotics to counter meningitis: the choice becomes harder," *Drug Therapy,* 12–13, November 1977.

Meissner, H. C., and Smith, A. L. "The current status of chloramphenicol," *Pediatrics,* 64: 348–56, 1979.

Mitsuhashi, S., et al., ed. *Drug Inactivating Enzymes and Antibiotic Resistance.* Springer-Verlag: New York, 1975.

Ray, S., et al. "Antibiotic cross-resistance patterns of Ambrodyl and Promazine resistant mutants," *British Journal of Experimental Pathology,* 61: 465–73, 1980.

Sprunt, K., et al. "Prevention of bacterial overgrowth," *Journal of Infectious Diseases,* 123: 1–10, 1971.

Weinswig, M. "Antibiotics Old and New," *Wisconsin Pharmacy Extension Bulletin,* 18: 1–4, 1975.

CHAPTER 5   WHAT HAPPENS WHEN I TAKE AN ANTIBIOTIC?

Andrews, M. *The Life That Lives on Man.* Taplinger Publishing Co.: New York, 1977.

Cluff, L. E., and Johnson III, J. E. *Clinical Concepts of Infectious Disease,* 2nd ed. Williams & Wilkins: Baltimore, 1978.

Drasar, B. S., and Hill, M. J. *Human Intestinal Flora.* Academic Press, Inc.: New York, 1974.

Drucker, D. B., and Jolly, M. "Sensitivity of oral microoganisms to antibiotics," *British Dental Journal,* 131: 442–45, 1971.

Evans, H. E., et al. "Factors influencing the establishment of the neonatal bacterial flora: I. The role of host factors," *Archives of Environmental Health,* 21: 514–19, 1970.

Fennery, A. R., et al. "A comparative study of gram negative aerobic bacilli in the faeces of babies born in hospital and at home," *Journal of Hygiene (Cambridge),* 84: 91–96, 1980.

Finland, M., and Bartmann, M. W., ed. *Bacterial Infections.* Springer-Verlag: Berlin, 1971.

Goldmann, D. A., et al. "Bacterial colonization of neonates admitted to an intensive care environment," *Journal of Pediatrics,* 93: 288–93, 1978.

Heimdahl, A., and Nord, C. E. "Effect of Phenoxymethylpenicillin and clindamycin on the oral, throat and faecal microflora of man," *Scandinavian Journal of Infectious Disease,* 11: 233–42, 1979.

Hirsch, D. C., et al. "Effect of oral tetracycline on the occurrence of tetracycline-resistant strains of *Escherichia coli* in the intestinal tract of humans," *Antimicrobial Agents and Chemotherapy,* 4: 69–71, 1973.

Long, S. S., and Swenson, R. M. "Development of anaerobic fecal flora in healthy newborn infants," *Journal of Pediatrics,* 91: 298–301, 1977.

Rosebury, T. *Life on Man.* Viking Press: New York, 1969.

————. *Microorganisms Indigenous to Man.* McGraw-Hill: New York, 1962.

Sprunt, K., et al. "Pharyngeal implantation of alpha hemolytic streptococci in neonates in an ICU," *Pediatric Research,* 11: 506–10, 1977.

Youmans, G. P., et al. *The Biologic and Clinical Basis of Infectious Diseases.* W. B. Saunders Company: Philadelphia, 1975.

CHAPTER 6   THE WHYS AND WHEREFORES OF RESISTANCE

Anonymous. "Community–acquired methicillin–resistant *Staphylococcus aureus*—Michigan," *Morbidity and Mortality Weekly Report,* 30: 185–87, 1981.

Asheshov, E. H. "The genetics of tetracycline resistance in Staphylococcus aureus," *Journal of General Microbiology,* 88: 132–40, 1975.

Crossley, K., et al. "An outbreak of infections caused by strains of *Staphylococcus aureus* resistant to methicillin and aminoglycosides," *Journal of Infectious Diseases,* 139: 273–87, 1979.

Gardner, P., et al. "Recovery of resistance (R) factors from a drug-free community," *Lancet,* 2: 774–76, 1969.

Hummel, R. P., et al. "Antibiotic resistance transfer from nonpathogenic to pathogenic bacteria," *Surgery,* 82: 382–85, 1977.

Musher, D. M., et al. "Selection of small colony variants of enterobacteriaceae by in vitro exposure to aminoglycosides," *Journal of Infectious Diseases,* 140: 209–13, 1979.

Petrocheilou, V., et al. "R-plasmid transfer in vivo in the absence of antibiotic selection pressure," *Antimicrobial Agents and Chemotherapy*, 10: 753–61, 1976.

Richards, H., and Datta, N. "Transposons and trimethoprim resistance," *British Medical Journal*, 282: 1118–19, 1981.

Roe, E., et al. "Transfer of antibiotic resistance between *Pseudomonas aeruginosa, Escherichia coli,* and other gram-negative bacilli in burns," *Lancet*, 1: 149–52, 1971.

Saah, A. J., et al. "Relative resistance to penicillin in the pneumococcus," *Journal of the American Medical Association*, 243: 1824–27, 1980.

Sato, G., et al. "Detection of conjugative R plasmids conferring chloramphenicol resistance in Escherichia coli isolated from domestic and feral pigeons and crows," *Zentralblatt Bakteriologie* (Original Article Series A), 241: 404–17, 1978.

Smith, D. H. "R factor infection of *Escherichia coli* lyophilized in 1946," *Journal of Bacteriology*, 94: 2071–75, 1967.

Sykes, R. B., and Richmond, M. H. "R factors, beta-lactamase, and carbenicillin resistant Pseudomonas aeruginosa," *Lancet*, 2: 342–45, 1971.

Widh, A., and Skold, O. "Ubiquity of R factor mediated antibiotic resistance in the healthy population," *Scandinavian Journal of Infectious Disease*, 9: 40–45, 1977.

Wray, C., et al. "Studies on the development of chloramphenicol resistance in Salmonella typhimurium," *Research in Veterinarian Science*, 18: 94–99, 1975.

CHAPTER 7   THE DEVELOPMENT OF RESISTANCE

Akiba, T., et al. "Studies on the mechanism of development of multi-drug resistant Shigella strain," *Nhoniji-shimpo*, No. 1866: 46–50, 1960.

Anonymous. "Spread of Haemophilus influenzae type b," *Lancet*, 1: 649, 1981.

Barber, M. "Methicillin-resistant staphylococci," *Journal of Clinical Pathology,* 14: 385–93, 1961.

Blackwell, C. C., and Feingold, D. S. "Frequency and some properties of clinical isolates of methicillin-resistant *Staphylococcus aureus,*" *American Journal of Clinical Pathology,* 64: 372–77, 1975.

Bulger, R. J. "A methicillin-resistant strain of Staphylococcus aureus," *Annals of Internal Medicine,* 67: 81–89, 1967.

Dean, H. F., et al. "Isolates of Pseudomonas aeruginosa from Australian hospitals having R-plasmid determined antibiotic resistance," *Medical Journal of Australia,* 2: 116–19, 1977.

Faden, H., et al. "Gentamicin-resistant Staphylococcus aureus. Emergence in an intensive care nursery," *Journal of the American Medical Association,* 241: 143–45, 1979.

Falkner, F. R., et al. "Cross infection in a surgical ward caused by Pseudomonas aeruginosa with transmissable resistance to gentamicin and tobramycin," *Journal of the Medical Association of Georgia,* 67: 22–25, 1978.

Finland, M. "Changing patterns of common bacterial pathogens to antimicrobial agents," *Annals of Internal Medicine,* 76: 1009–13, 1972.

Follow-up on multiple-antibiotic resistant pneumococci—South Africa, *Morbidity and Mortality Weekly Report,* 27: 1, 1978.

Grunt, J., and Krcmery, V. "Multiple drug resistance in staphylococci: An analysis of all nation computer processed data," *Zentralblatt für Bakteriologie* (Original Article Series A), 234: 14–20, 1976.

Hosseini, H. "Bacterial sensitivity to antibiotics," *Current Therapeutic Research,* 11: 397–405, 1969.

Iannini, P. B., et al. "Multidrug-resistant Proteus rettgeri: an emerging problem," *Annals of Internal Medicine,* 85: 1616–24, 1976.

Kaplan, S. L., et al. "Effect of prior antibiotics on the susceptibility of *Hemophilus influenzae* Type b to ampicillin," *Pediatrics,* 67: 269–71, 1981.

Maness, M. J., and Sparling, P. F. "Multiple antibiotic resistance due to a single mutation in Neisseria gonorrhoeae," *Journal of Infectious Diseases,* 128: 321–30, 1973.

McConnell, M. M., et al. "The value of plasmid studies in the epidemiology of infections due to drug resistant Salmonella wien," *Journal of Infectious Diseases,* 139: 179–89, 1979.

Murphy, D., and Todd, J. "Treatment of ampicillin-resistant Haemophilus influenzae in soft tissue infections with high doses of ampicillin," *Journal of Pediatrics,* 94: 983–87, 1979.

Nelson, J. D. "Should ampicillin be abandoned for the treatment of Haemophilus influenzae disease?" *Journal of the American Medical Association,* 229: 322–24, 1976.

O'Brien, T. F., et al. "International surveillance of prevalence of antibiotic resistance," *Journal of Antimicrobial Chemotherapy (Supplement C),* 3: 59–66, 1977.

Ochai, K., et al. "Studies on the inheritance of drug resistance between Shigella strain and E. coli strains," *Nhoniji-shimpo,* No. 1861: 34–36, 1959.

Shanson, D. C., et al. "Outbreak of hospital infection with a strain of Staphylococcus aureus resistant to gentamicin and methicillin," *Lancet,* 2: 1347–48, 1976.

Sieber, W. T., et al. "Resistance to gentamicin: A growing concern," *Southern Medical Journal,* 70: 289–93, 1977.

Siegel, J. D., and McCracken, Jr., G. H. "Sepsis neonatorum," *New England Journal of Medicine,* 304: 642–47, 1981.

Smith, A. L. "Antiobiotics and invasive Haemophilus influenzae," *New England Journal of Medicine,* 29: 1329–30, 1976.

Smith, H. W. "Mutants of Klebsiella pneumoniae resistant to several antibiotics," *Nature,* 259: 307–8, 1976.

Southern, Jr., P. M., and Sanford, J. P. "Meningococcal meningitis—Suboptimal response to cephalothin therapy," *New England Journal of Medicine,* 280: 1163–64, 1969.

Suenderhauf, U., et al. "Prevalence and characterization of resistance to gentamicin in Gram-negative bacteria," *Microbios,* 17: 221–30, 1976.

Thiemke, W. A., and Nathan, D. M. "Simultaneous nosocomial outbreaks caused by multiply resistant Klebsiella pneumoniae types 2 and 30," *Journal of Clinical Microbiology,* 8: 769–71, 1978.

Thomas, W. J., and McReynolds, J. W. "Haemophilus influenzae resistant to penicillin," *Lancet,* 2: 13–16, 1971.

Vchiyama, N., et al. "Meningitis due to Haemophilus influenzae resistant to ampicillin and chloramphenicol," *Journal of Pediatrics,* 97: 421–24, 1980.

Watanabe, T. "Infective heredity of multiple drug resistance in bacteria," *Bacteriology Reviews,* 27: 87–103, 1963.

Yogev, R. "Use of trimethoprim-sulfamethoxazole against Haemophilus influenzae," *Journal of Pediatrics,* 96: April 1980.

CHAPTER 8   INAPPROPRIATE USE

Anonymous. "Antibiotic antagonism and synergy," *Lancet,* 2: 80–82, 1978.

Anonymous. "FDA seeks to ban Ilosone[R]" *Pediatric Alert,* 4: 77–78, 1979.

Anonymous. "When the culture is negative—cool it," *Emergency Medicine,* January 1977.

Bartlett, R. C., et al. "Quality assurance of Gram-stained direct smears," *American Journal of Clinical Pathology,* 72: 984–90, 1979.

Beckstrom, D., and Wang, R. I. H. "Surgical use of prophylactic antibiotics," *Drug Therapy,* 27–35: May 1977.

DuPont, H. L., et al. "Antimicrobial susceptibility of enterotoxigenic Escherichia coli," *Journal of Antimicrobial Chemotherapy,* 4: 100–10, 1978.

Erickson, S. H., et al. "The use of drugs for unlabeled indications," *Journal of the American Medical Association* 243: 1543–46, 1980.

Fekety, Jr., F. R. "The rational use of antibiotics," *Hospital Formulary,* January 1977, pp. 26–27, 31–32.

Garrod, L. G., and Waterworth, P. M. "Tests of bacterial sensitivity to drugs," *Disease a Month,* July 1971.

Hermans, P. E. "General principles of antimicrobial therapy," *Mayo Clinic Proceedings,* 52: 603–10, 1977.

Hill, C., et al. "Prophylactic cefazolin versus placebo in total hip replacement," *Lancet,* 1: 795–97, 1981.

Hirschmann, J. V., and Innue, T. S. "Antibiotic Prophylaxis: A critique of recent trials," *Reviews of Infectious Disease,* 2: 1–23, 1980.

Jogerst, G. J., and Dippe, S. E. "Antibiotic use among medical specialities in a community hospital," *Journal of the American Medical Association,* 245: 842–46, 1981.

Kunin, C. M., and Efron, H. Y. "Audits of antimicrobial usage, Veterans Administration Ad Hoc Interdisciplinary Committee on Antimicrobial Usage," *Journal of the American Medical Association,* 237: 1001–7, 1134–37, 1241–45, 1366–69, 1481–84, 1605–8, 1723–25, 1859–60, 1967–70, 1977.

Latorraca, R., and Martins, R. "Surveillance of antibiotic use in a community hospital," *Journal of the American Medical Association,* 242: 2585–87, 1979.

LaViolett, S. "System slashes surveillance time," *Modern Healthcare,* July 1979, p. 30.

Loening-Baucke, V. A., et al. "A placebo-controlled trial of cephalexin therapy in the ambulatory management of patients with cystic fibrosis," *Journal of Pediatrics,* 95: 630–37, 1979.

Pien, F. D., et al. "Antibiotic use in a small community hospital," *Western Journal of Medicine,* 130: 498–502, 1979.

Quinn, E. L. "Prevention of bacterial infection by non-immunologic methods," in *Current Concepts of Infectious Disease,* ed. E. W. Hook, et al. John Wiley & Sons: New York, 1977.

Roberts, A. W., and Visconti, J. A. "The rational and irrational use of systemic antimicrobial drugs," *American Journal of Hospital Pharmacy,* 29: 828–34, 1972.

Schonholtz, G. J., et al. "Wound sepsis in orthopedic surgery," *Journal of Bone and Joint Surgery,* 44 A: 1548–52, 1962.

Shapiro, M., et al. "Use of antimicrobial drugs in a general hospital. II. Analysis of patterns of use," *Journal of Infectious Diseases,* 139: 698–711, 1979.

Yogev, R., et al. "Effect of TMP-SMX on nasopharyngeal carriage of ampicillin-sensitive and ampicillin-resistant Hemophilus influenzae type B," *Journal of Pediatrics,* 93: 394–97, 1978.

CHAPTER 9   GETTING SICK IN THE HOSPITAL?

Bacterial Diseases Division, Bureau of Epidemiology, Public Health Service, CDC Atlanta, Ga. "Nosocomial gastrointestinal illness in neonates—Houston, Texas," Internal memo No. EPI-76-14-1.

Bennett, J. V. "Incidence and nature of endemic and epidemic nosocomial infections," in *Hospital Infections,* ed. J. V. Bennett and P. S. Brachman. Little, Brown and Co.: Boston, 1979.

———. "Nosocomial infections due to Pseudomonas," *Journal of Infectious Diseases (Supplement),* 130: 1–166, 1974.

———, and Brachman, P. S., eds. *Hospital Infections.* Little, Brown and Co.: Boston, 1979.

Bradley, H. E., et al. "Tolerance in Staphylococcus aureus," *Lancet,* 1: 150, 1979.

Bryan, C. S., et al. "Plasmid-mediated antibiotic resistance in a changing hospital environment," *American Journal of Infection Control,* 8: 65–71, 1980.

Craig, W. A., et al. "Hospital use of antimicrobial drugs," *Annals of Internal Medicine,* 89 (Part 2): 793–95, 1978.

Dixon, R. E. "Nosocomial infection. A continuing problem," *Postgraduate Medicine,* 62: 95–109, 1977.

Eickhoff, T. C. "General comments on the study on the efficacy of nosocomial infection control (SENIC Project)," *American Journal of Epidemiology,* 111: 465–69, 1980.

Finland, M. "Emergence of antibiotic resistance in hospitals, 1935–1975," *Reviews of Infectious Disease,* 1: 4–21, 1980.

Fontaine, T. D., and Hoadley, A. W. "Transferable drug resistance associated with coliforms isolated from hospital and domestic sewage," *Health and Laboratory Science,* 13: 238–45, 1976.

Haley, R. W., and Shachtman, R. H. "The emergence of infection surveillance and control programs in US hospitals: An assessment, 1976," *American Journal of Epidemiology,* 111: 574–91, 1980.

Jonsson, M. "Antibiotic resistance and R factors in gram negative bacteria," *Scandinavian Journal of Infectious Disease, Supplement 5,* 1977: 1–103.

Jung, R. C., and Aaronson, J. "Death following inhalation of mercury vapor at home," *Western Journal of Medicine,* 132: 539–42, 1980.

Kunin, C. M. "Problems of antibiotic usage: Definitions, causes and proposed solutions," *Annals of Internal Medicine,* 89 (Part 2): 802–5, 1978.

————, and Efron, H. Y. chair and vice-chair, respectively, Veterans Administration Ad Hoc Interdisciplinary Advisory Committee on Antimicrobial Drug Usage, "Guidelines for Peer Review," *Journal of the Amercian Medical Association,* 237: 1001–8, 1977.

Maki, D. G. "Control of colonization and transmission of pathogenic bacteria in the hospital," *Annals of Internal Medicine,* 89 (Part 2): 777–80, 1978.

Myclotte, J. M., and Beam, Jr., T. R. "Comparison of community-acquired and nosocomial pneumococcal bacteremia," *American Review of Respiratory Disease,* 123: 265–68, 1981.

Olexy, V. M., et al. "Hospital isolates of Serratia marcescens transferring ampicillin, carbenicillin, and gentamicin resistance to other gram-negative bacteria including Pseudomonas aeruginosa," *Antimicrobial Agents and Chemotherapy,* 15: 93–100, 1979.

Ridley, M., and Phillips, I. *The Therapeutic Use of Antibiotics in Hospital Practice.* E. S. Livingstone: London, 1966.

Rosendal, K., et al. "Antibiotic policy and spread of Staphylococcus aureus strains in the Danish hospitals, 1969–1974," *Acta Pathologica Microbiologica Scandinavia,* 85: 143–52, 1977.

Schaberg, D. R., et al. "An outbreak of nosocomial infection due to multiply resistant Serratia marcescens: Evidence of interhospital spread," *Journal of Infectious Diseases,* 134: 181–87, 1976.

Shapiro, M., et al. "Use of antimicrobial drugs in general hospitals," *New England Journal of Medicine,* 301: 351–55, 1979.

Warren, J. W., et al. "Antibiotic irrigation and catheter-associated urinary tract infections," *New England Journal of Medicine,* 299: 570–73, 1978.

Wenzel, R. P., et al. "Development of a statewide program for surveillance and reporting of hospital-acquired infections," *Journal of Infectious Diseases,* 140: 741–46, 1979.

Young, V. M., et al. "Origin of infection in acute nonlymphocytic leukemia: Significance of hospital acquisition of potential pathogens," *Annals of Internal Medicine,* 77: 707–14, 1972.

CHAPTER 10   ANTIBIOTICS AT THE FEEDLOT

Anonymous. "Infectious drug resistance," *New England Journal of Medicine,* 275: 277, 1966.

Anonymous. "Salmonellosis—An unhappy turn of events," *Lancet,* 1: 1009–10, 1979.

Anthan, G. "Ban on antibiotics in animal feed could be a boon for family farms," *Des Moines Register,* February 1, 1979.

Baker, R., et al. "Phage type/biotype groups of Salmonella typhimurium in Scotland 1974–6: variation during spread of epidemic clones," *Journal of Hygiene (Cambridge),* 84: 115–25, 1980.

Bird, H. R. "One man's meat," *The Sciences* (letter), 19: 2–3, 1979.

Dingell, J. D., House of Representatives, U. S. Congress, "Animal feeds: Effects of antibiotics," *Science,* 208: 1069, September 5, 1980.

Dixon, B. "Antibiotics redux," *The Sciences,* 20: 28, 1980.

Farris, A. S., et al. "Antibiotic resistance and transferable antibiotic resistant Escherichia coli isolated from calves on a modern farm with therapeutic problems and unsatisfactory management conditions," *Nordic Veterinary Medicine,* 31: 20–24, 1979.

Fein, D., et al. "Matching of antibiotic resistance patterns of Escherichia coli of farm families and their animals," *Journal of Infectious Diseases,* 130: 274–301, 1974.

Franklin, A., and Glatthard, V. "R-factor mediated antibiotic resistance in E. coli strains isolated from piglets in Sweden," *Zentralblatt Bakteriologie* (Original Article Series A), 238: 208–15, 1977.

Gunby, P. "No resolution on question of antibiotics in feed," *Journal of the American Medical Association,* 243: 1618, 1980.

Hays, V. W. "Effectiveness of feed additive usage of antibacterial agents in swine and poultry," Paper for OTA, U. S. Congress, 1978 Tables 41, 42 & 43, Table 14.

Howells, C. H. L., and Joynson, D. H. M. "Possible role of animal feeding-stuffs in spread of antibiotic-resistant intestinal coliforms," *Lancet,* 1: 156–57, 1975.

Jukes, T. H. "Antibiotics in feeds," *Science* (letter), 204: 8, 1979.

———. "Antibiotics, resistance, and animal growth: Another view," *The Sciences,* 20: 24–27, 1980.

Levy, S. B., et al. "Changes in intestinal flora of farm personnel after introduction of a tetracycline-supplemented feed on a farm," *New England Journal of Medicine,* 295: 583–88, 1976.

Marshall, E. "Health committee investigates farm drugs," *Science,* 209: 481–82, 1980.

———. "Scientists quit antibiotics panel at CAST," *Science,* 203: 732–33, 1979.

Novick, R. P. "Antibiotics: Use in animal feed," *Science* (letter), 204: 908, 1979.

———. "Antibiotics: Wonder drugs or chicken feed," *The Sciences,* 19: 14–17, 1979.

Office of Technology Assessment, *Drugs in Livestock Feed*, Vol. I, Technical Report, Washington, D.C., 1979.

Pohl, P. "Relationship between antibiotic feeding in animals and emergence of bacterial resistance in man," *Journal of Antimicrobial Chemotherapy*, (Supplement C), 3: 67–72, 1977.

Smith, H. W., and Tucker, J. F. "Further observations on the effect of feeding diets containing avoparcin, bacitracin and sodium arsenilate on the colonization of the alimentary tract of poultry by salmonella organisms," *Journal of Hygiene (Cambridge)*, 84: 137–41, 1980.

Sogaard, H. "The incidence of antibiotic resistance among coliform bacteria isolated from food," *Acta Veterinaria Scandinavia*, 17: 271–78, 1976.

CHAPTER 11   NONANTIBIOTIC REMEDIES

Ad Hoc Committee on the Use of Antibiotics in Dermatology, "Systemic antibiotics for treatment of acne vulgaris efficacy and safety," *Archives of Dermatology*, 111: 1630–36, 1975.

Colaert, J., et al. "Antimicrobial susceptibility of Vibrio cholerae from Zaire and Rwanda," *Lancet*, 2: 849, 1979.

DuPont, H. L., et al. "Prevention of traveler's diarrhea (Emporiatric enteritis)," *Journal of the American Medical Association*, 243: 237–41, 1980.

Fisher, E. J. "Traveler's diarrhea: New Concepts," *Journal of Occupational Medicine*, 23: 277–80, 1981.

Freinkel, R. K. "Pathogenesis of acne vulgaris," *New England Journal of Medicine*, 280: 1161–63, 1969.

Kaijser, B. "Pneumococcal infections and the possible need for a vaccine," *Scandinavian Journal of Infectious Disease*, 11: 25–33, 1979.

Kasper, D. L., et al. "Protective efficacy of immunization with capsular antigen against experimental infection with Bacteroides fragilis," *Journal of Infectious Diseases*, 140: 724–31, 1979.

McCracken, Jr., G. H. "Commentary," *Journal of Pediatrics,* 94: 987, 1979.

Mhalu, F. S., et al. "Rapid emergence of El Tor Vibrio cholerae resistant to antimicrobial agents during first six months of fourth cholera epidemic in Tanzania," *Lancet,* 1: 345–47, 1979.

Mills, E. L., et al. "The chemiluminescence response and bactericidal activity of polymorphonuclear neutrophils from newborns and their mothers," *Pediatrics,* 63: 429–34, 1979.

Muster, A. M., et al. "The effect of antibiotics on cell-mediated immunity," *Surgery,* 81: 692–95, 1977.

Pennington, J. E. "Lipopolysaccharide pseudomonas vaccine: efficacy against pulmonary infection with Pseudomonas aeuruginosa," *Journal of Infectious Diseases,* 140: 73–80, 1979.

Pochi, P. E. "Antibiotics in acne," *New England Journal of Medicine,* 294: 43–44, 1976.

Pollack, M. *"Pseudomonas aeruginosa* exotoxin A," *New England Journal of Medicine,* 302: 1360–61, 1980.

Rosenberg, M. L., et al. "Epidemic diarrhea at Crater Lake from enterotoxigenic Escherichia coli," *Annals of Internal Medicine,* 86: 714–18, 1977.

Scotland, S. M., et al. "The occurrence of plasmids carrying genes for both enterotoxin production and drug resistance in Escherichia coli of human origin," *Journal of Hygiene (Cambridge),* 83: 531–37, 1979.

Shuster, S. "13-Cis-retinoic acid for acne," *Lancet,* 2: 50, 1979.

Swinyer, L. J., et al. "Topical agents alone in acne: A blind assessment study," *Journal of the American Medical Association,* 243: 1640–43, 1980.

Taylor, M. R. H., et al. "Simple and effective measures for control of enteric cross-infection in a children's hospital," *Lancet,* 2: 865–67, 1979.

Tong, Y. H. "Antimicrobials with immunosuppressive potential," *Medical Journal of Australia,* 1: 444–45, 1978 (letter).

Volman, H. B. "Infants of low birth weight," *British Medical Journal,* 2: 1431–32, 1979.

Willems, J. S., et al. "Cost effectiveness of vaccination against pneumococcal pneumonia," *New England Journal of Medicine,* 313: 553–59, 1980.

CHAPTER 12   NEW APPROACHES TO CONTROLLING BACTERIA

Battett, F. F., et al. "The effect of three cord-care regiments on bacterial colonization of normal, newborn infants," *Journal of Pediatrics,* 94: 796–800, 1979.

Bibel, D. J., et al. "Skin flora maps: A tool in the study of cutaneous ecology," *Journal of Investigative Dermatology,* 67: 265–69, 1976.

Black, R. E., et al. "Handwashing to prevent diarrhea in day-care centers," *American Journal of Epidemiology,* 113: 445–51, 1981.

Fitzgerald, Jr., R. H. "Preoperative surgical skin disinfection," *Journal of the American Medical Association,* 242: 2889, 1979.

General Discussion, "Symposium on nonchemotherapeutic Approaches to Control of Staphylococcal Infection," Bulletin of the New York Academy of Medicine, 44: 1227–36, 1968.

Kominos, S. D., et al. "Dietary controls for pseudomonas infections," *Hospital Infection Control,* 2: 73–75, 1975.

Lister, J. "Aseptic technique and adjunctive treatment of the surgical field," *British Medical Journal,* 4: 246, 1867.

Noble, W. C., and Willie, J. A. "Interactions between antibiotic-producing and nonproducing staphylococci in skin-surface and sub-surface models," *British Journal of Experimental Pathology,* 61: 339–43, 1980.

Orfuss, A. J., et al. "General discussion: Symposium on Nonchemotherapeutic Approaches to Control of Staphylococcal Infection," A. L. Florman, moderator, in *Bulletin of the New York Academy of Medicine (2nd Series),* 44: 1227–36, 1968.

Pollock, A. V. "Surgical wound sepsis," *Lancet*, 2: 1283–86, 1979.

Report of the European Organization of Research on Treatment of Cancer, "Protective isolation and antimicrobial decontamination in patients with high susceptibility to infection: A prospective study of gnotobiotic care in acute leukemia patients," *Infection*, 5: 107–14, 1977.

Selwyn, S. "Natural antibiosis among skin bacteria as a primary defence against infection," *British Journal of Dermatology*, 93: 487–95, 1975.

CHAPTER 13   REACTIVATING THE BODY'S OWN NATURAL
                DEFENSES

Akonkhai, V. F., et al. "Failure of pneumococcal vaccine in children with sickle cell disease," *New England Journal of Medicine*, 301: 26–27, 1979.

Anonymous. "Pseudomonas vaccine reduces burn mortality," *Medical World News*, 19: 40–41, 1978.

Anonymous. "Wide-spectrum antiserum cuts bacteremia deaths," *Medical World News*, 19: 44, 1978.

Belsheim, J., et al. "Tetracyclines and host defense mechanisms: Interference with leukocyte chemotaxis," *Scandinavian Journal of Infectious Disease*, 11: 141–45, 1979.

Broome, C. V., et al. "Pneumococcal disease after pneumococcal vaccination," *New England Journal of Medicine*, 303: 549–52, 1980.

Cluff, L. E. "Recovery from Infection," in *Clinical Concepts of Infectious Disease*, pp. 168–77.

Fiumara, M. K., and Waterman, G. E. "Statewide geriatric immunization program with polyvalent pneumococcal vaccine," *Current Therapeutic Research*, 25: 185–92, 1979.

Guckian, J. C., et al. "Role of opsonins in recovery from experimental pneumonia," *Journal of Infectious Diseases*, 175: 175–90, 1980.

Hammond, W. P., and Dale, D. C. "Infections in the compromised host," *Hospital Medicine,* May 1978, pp. 87–116.

Jones, J., et al. "Controlled trials of a polyvalent pseudomonas vaccine in burns," *Lancet,* 2: 977–83, 1979.

Patrick, K. M., and Woolley, F. R. "A cost-benefit analysis of immunization for pneumococcal pneumonia," *Journal of the American Medical Association,* 245: 473–77, 1981.

CHAPTER 14   CONCLUSION

Neu, H. C., and Howrey, S. P. "Testing the physician's knowledge of antibiotic usage," *New England Journal of Medicine,* 293: 1291–95, 1975.

Sack, R. B. "Prophylactic antibiotics? The individual versus the community," *New England Journal of Medicine,* 300: 1107–8, 1979.

Self, S. B. "Gold dust: Great new germ killer," *Science Digest,* 28: 74–77, 1950.

Simmons, H. E. "An overview of public policy and infectious diseases," *Annals of Internal Medicine,* 89 (Part 2): 821–25, 1978.

Stimson, Jr., T. E. "Penicillin: New rival of the sulfas," *Science Digest,* 14: 31–33, 1943.

Glossary

A Lexicon of Antibiotic
Related Words & Terms

Actinomycetes: a group of fungi of the genus *Actinomyces* including *A. antibioticus* from which a number of antibiotics have been isolated.

Adenitis: an inflammation of the lymph nodes.

AHA: abbreviation for the American Hospital Association.

Allergenic: capable of provoking an allergic response.

Aminoglycoside: a group of injectable antibiotics which have the ability to resist degradation by penicillinases.

Amoxicillin: a partially synthesized (semisynthetic) derivative of the penicillin family with increased oral absorption and urinary excretion that can be taken by mouth.

Ampicillin: an injectable penicillin with the same general spectrum of activity as amoxicillin.

Amplification: the process by which a DNA molecule makes many copies of a particular gene and thereby increases the number of molecules generated by that gene sequence.

Anaerobic: able to live in the absence of oxygen; cf. obligate anaerobe, an organism requiring the absence of oxygen in order to live.

Antagonism: the phenomenon by which one antibiotic interferes with the therapeutic activity of another.

Antibiosis: the phenomenon by which one type of microorganism inhibits the growth or survival of another, usually through production of "natural" antibiotics (see *Bacterial interference*).

Antibiotic: any natural or synthetic chemical able to affect the survival of microorganisms through inhibiting their growth or killing them.

Antibiotic resistance: the ability of a microorganism to survive exposure to an otherwise detrimental antibiotic.

Anticoagulant: an agent having the ability to prevent the clotting of blood.

Antimicrobic susceptibility test: a procedure used to measure the vulnerability of a given bacterium to the inhibiting or killing effect of a specific concentration of an antibiotic.

Antisepsis: the process by which bacterial colonization is prevented.

Aplastic anemia: an often irreversible condition characterized by reduction of circulating red blood cells due to the destruction of centers of production in the bone marrow.

Aureomycin: a proprietary name for chlortetracycline.

Bacitracin: a topical antibiotic active primarily against gram-positive organisms.

Bacterial interference: syn. antibiosis.

Bacteriostatic: controlling or limiting the growth of bacteria.

Bacteriotoxic: toxic to and thereby lethal for bacteria.

Bacteroides: an anaerobic, gram-negative genus of bacteria often associated with infections of the brain; the most common genus of bacteria isolated from the intestine or vagina.

Beta-lactam: the ring structure of penicillin and cephalosporin molecules.

Bifidus (literally, "two tailed"): a species of bacteria commonly found on the skin (see *Diphtheroids*).

Broad-spectrum antibiotic: an antibiotic active against a wide range of disease-causing bacteria.

Campylobacter: a genus of gram-negative bacteria.

Carbenicillin: a partially synthesized penicillin partially effective against *Pseudomonas* and *Proteus* species of bacteria; it is ineffective against *Staphylococcus*.

CAST: abbreviation for the industry-sponsored Council for Agricultural Science and Technology.

CDC: abbreviation for the federal Center for Disease Control in Atlanta, Georgia.

Cephalosporins: a group of modern, beta-lactam antibiotics particularly effective in treating penicillin-resistant infections, particularly those caused by gram-negative organisms like *E. coli, Klebsiella,* or *Proteus mirabilis* organisms.

Chloramphenicol: a potent and toxic antibiotic particularly effective in treating typhoid fever and meningitis.

Chloromycetin: the proprietary name for chloramphenicol.

Chlortetracycline: a golden-colored antibiotic isolated from *Streptomyces aureofacens* with broad activity against a wide spectrum of microorganisms; its proprietary name is Aureomycin.

Cholera: a usually severe, acute infectious disease caused by *Vibrio cholerae* that is characterized by diarrhea, cramps, and collapse. The extreme loss of bodily fluids and salts (electrolytes) that accompanies it can lead to death unless replacement is rapidly achieved.

Chromosomal genes: in bacteria, that genetic information carried on the bacteria's own chromosome (cf. *Plasmids*).

Clostridium: a genus of anaerobic bacteria including *C. botulinum* and *C. difficile* capable of producing extraordinarily poisonous toxins and hence serious disease or death in infected hosts.

Cloxacillin: an orally administered, penicillinase-resistant penicillin that is particularly well absorbed.

Coliforms: the group of gram-negative bacteria including *Escherichia coli* that are normally found in the intestinal tract.

Colonization: the seeding and outgrowth of a bacterium in an area previously uninhabited by that organism.

Commensal (literally, "at the same table"): referring to organisms that are able to live from the same subsistence base without interfering with each other.

Conjugation: the mating process in bacteria by which genetic information is exchanged between two genetically distinct organisms.

Dicloxacillin: an orally administered, penicillinase-resistant penicillin (cf. *Cloxacillin*).

Diphtheroids: a group of bacteria related to the propionibacteria that are common inhabitants of the skin; so named because of their resemblance to the organism that causes diphtheria, *Corynebacterium diphtheriae.*

Elective: a procedure or operation in which the underlying condition does not require immediate attention.

Endocarditis: an inflammation of the lining of the heart, usually confined to the external lining of the valves.

Enteritis: an inflammation of the lining of the intestine.

Erythromycin: an orally effective derivative of *Streptomyces* often used prophylactically to prevent blood-borne infection with *Streptococcus* strains capable of producing endocarditis.

Escherichia: a ubiquitous genus of bacteria inhabiting the human intestinal tract that is capable of causing enteritis and urinary tract infections.

Escherichia coli: (abbrev. *E. coli*) the most common species of *Escherichia,* now recognized as a potential pathogen that predominates the human intestinal flora.

ETEC: an abbreviation for enterotoxigenic *E. coli,* a toxin-producing strain of this common intestinal bacterium.

Excretion: the release of waste products; in bacteriology, the discharge of bacteria or bacterial products in the urine or feces.

Flora: the combined total of kinds and types of microorganisms at a specific anatomical site.

Gantrisin: proprietary name for the sulfa drug sulfisoxazole commonly used for treating urinary tract infections.

Genome: the male or female contribution to the genetic makeup of an individual organism; in bacteria, the chromosomal genes of a given organism.

Gentamicin: a broad-spectrum aminoglycoside antibiotic active against both gram-negative and gram-positive bacteria.

Gonococcus (literally, "little berry"): usually, the organism that causes gonorrhea, *Neisseria gonococcus* (syn. *N. gonorrhoeae*); any organism in the genus.

Gramicidin: an early, toxic antibiotic effective against gram-positive bacteria.

Gram-negative: bacteria that lose the primary Gram stain (a violet-colored chemical) and pick up a counterstain, usually carbolfuchsin or safranine.

Gram-positive: retaining the color of the gentian violet stain in Gram's method of staining.

Gram stain (cf. Gram's method): a process developed by the Danish physician Hans C. J. Gram (1853–1938) for staining bacteria; the stain used to identify broad classes of bacteria based on their cell coat or capsule's ability to pick up specific dyes.

Hemophilus: a genus of small, gram-negative bacilli often the cause of penicillin-resistant infections in children; cf. *H. influenzae* type b, a major cause of respiratory and middle ear infections and meningitis.

Iatrogenesis (literally, "caused by a physician"): physician-induced disease or injury.

Inhibition: the limiting or cessation of growth and/or division of a bacterium by an antibiotic short of direct killing (see *Bacteriostatic*).

Invasive: having the ability to penetrate and spread beyond the initial focus of infection.

Kanamycin: an injectable antibiotic frequently used against serious gram-positive or gram-negative rod infections of childhood.

Klebsiella: a genus of gram-negative, encapsulated bacteria frequently associated with upper respiratory and urinary tract infections.

Lactamase: an enzyme capable of splitting off the beta-lactam ring.

Lactobacillus: a common, lactic acid-producing bacterium found in the mouth, intestinal tract, and vagina.

Meninges: the three membranes that surround the brain and spinal cord.

Meningitis: an inflammation of the meninges of the brain.

Metabolism: the chemical and physical reactions that take place in an organism to produce energy or transform chemicals.

Methicillin: a semisynthethic penicillin that is resistant to enzymatic breakdown by penicillinases.

Metronidazole: a potent antibiotic effective against many anaerobic bacteria, used as the treatment of choice against *Trichomonas* infections; it is mutagenic and carcinogenic in animals.

MIC: abbreviation for minimum inhibitory concentration, the lowest concentration in an antimicrobic susceptibility test that limits the growth of bacteria.

Micrococcus: a genus of bacteria commonly found on the skin.

Microflora: the microscopic organisms that inhabit a specific anatomical site (see *Flora*).

Mycelia: the microscopic roots of a fungus.

Natural selection: the evolutionary process by which organisms better adapted to reproduce in a given environment predominate.

Neurotoxic: poisonous to nervous tissue or cells.

Nitrofurans: a potent group of antibiotics used in treating urinary tract infections (see *Nitrofurantoin*).

Nitrofurantoin: a nitrofuran antibiotic used for treating bladder and kidney infections.

Nitrofurazone: a synthetic antibiotic for topical application in some skin diseases.

NNIS: abbreviation for National Nosocomial Infection Study.

Nonpathogenic: incapable of producing disease.

Nosocomial (literally, "a place where diseases are cared for"): of or pertaining to a hospital or infirmary.

Nosocomial infection: an infection acquired in a hospital.

NRC: abbreviation for National Research Council.

Otitis media: inflammation of the middle ear.

Parenteral(ly): located outside the intestines; cf. *parenteral injection.*

Parenteral injection: introduction of substances to the body by any route other than through the alimentary canal.

Pathogenic: capable of producing disease.

Pelvic inflammatory disease: an invasive disease of the pelvic organs, usually involving the oviducts and uterus and commonly caused by gonococci.

Penicillin: the first relatively nontoxic antibiotic to find clinical usefulness against gram-positive organisms; isolated by Sir Alexander Fleming in 1927 from the *Penicillium* mold.

Penicillinase: an enzyme produced by many bacteria able to break down the penicillin molecule by splitting off the lactam ring.

Penicillium: the genus of mold from which penicillin was first isolated.

Pharyngitis: an inflammation of the pharynx or throat.

Pili: the surface extrusions of some forms of bacteria.

Plasmids: the composite of replicating and resistance genes that together comprise the self-reproducing satellite chromosomes that infect some bacteria (see *R factor*).

Pneumococcus (literally, "berry of the lung"): a gram-positive bacterium that usually occurs in pairs and includes seventy-five different serotypes capable of causing respiratory and other infections.

Pneumonia: an inflammation of the lungs caused primarily by bacteria, viruses, and chemical irritants, but having over fifty different possible causes.

Polymyxin: a potent, basic polypeptide antibiotic capable of producing neurotoxicity that is often used against infections caused by *Pseudomonas.*

PPNG: abbreviation for penicillinase-producing *Neisseria gonnorrhoeae.*

Prontosil: an early antibiotic.

Prophylaxis (literally, "warding off disease"): preventing infection through the use of chemotherapeutic agents, notably antibiotics.

Propionibacterium: a genus of bacteria that is uniquely associated with infections of implanted heart valves; a species (*P. acnes*) is associated with acne lesions.

Proteus: a major genus of Enterobacteriaceae commonly found in wound and burn infections.

Pseudomonas: the genus of small, motile, gram-negative bacilli that include *Pseudomonas aeruginosa,* a gram-negative bacterium capable of causing urinary tract infections and otitis media.

Puerperal fever: a blood poisoning (septicemia) following childbirth.

Pyocins: bacteriostatic substances isolated from *Pseudomonas* species.

Pyoderma: a deep infection of soft tissues, usually caused by *Staphylococcus.*

R factor: a genetic factor in bacteria which controls resistance to certain antibiotic drugs capable of being spread from one organism to another, thereby facilitating the conversion of nonpathogenic bacteria to antibiotic-resistant reservoirs of genes that can form the focus of a potential epidemic of antibiotic-resistant, pathogenic organisms (cf. *resistance transfer factor*).

Replica plate(s): a Petri dish containing nutrient agar onto which a pattern of bacteria is implanted from a like dish in precisely the same orientation; two Petri dishes in which colonies of bacteria are distributed identically.

Replication: the act of replicating or reproducing one cell from another (synonym: *division*).

Resistance transfer factor: part of an *R factor*.

RTF: abbreviation for resistance transfer factor; also, those genes on a plasmid responsible for permitting self-reproduction.

Salmonella: a gram-negative bacterium causing mild to severe gastroenteritis, occasionally leading to death.

Salvarsan: an arsenical preparation developed by Paul Ehrlich for the treatment of syphilis.

Selection pressure: the forces that lead to the survival of one type of organism over another.

Semisterile: the partial absence of bacteria, usually brought about by agents that drastically reduce the overall number of organisms.

SENIC: abbreviation for Study of the Efficacy of Nosocomial Infection Control.

Septic: pertaining to pathogenic bacteria or their products, e.g., toxins.

Septicemia: the presence of pathogenic organisms in the blood.

Septic phlebitis: an inflammation of the venous blood vessels of the leg accompanied by the presence of pathogenic bacteria.

Shigella: a genus of gram-negative bacteria that causes intestinal disease ranging from mild diarrhea to dysentery.

Spectinomycin: an aminocyclitol antibiotic particularly useful in treating acute gonorrhea infections caused by penicillin-resistant gonococci.

Staphylococcus: a genus of micrococci comprised of gram-positive bacteria, including many pathogenic species that cause suppurative infections and that can release toxins destructive to tissues and cells.

Sterile: the complete absence of viable bacteria.

Streptococcus: the genus of gram-positive bacteria, usually occurring in chains, that includes species pathogenic to humans, especially children.

Subtherapeutic: the use of drugs at doses below those needed to treat disease.

Sulfa: abbreviation for sulfanilamide or other sulfonamide antibiotics.

Sulfanilamide: (paraaminobenzenesulfonamide) an early toxic antibiotic superseded by the more effective sulfonamides; an antibiotic used to treat urinary infections.

Sulfonamides: a group of compounds made from amides of sulfanilic acid (sulfanilamide) that have bacteriostatic properties.

Superinfection: the overgrowth of bacteria, yeast, or fungi differing in kind from an initial infecting organism, usually following protracted treatment with antibiotics.

Surveillance: the use of review procedures intended to detect the occurrence and extent of episodes of infection; the sum total of all of the steps taken to chart the occurrence of specific bacterial infections in a given setting.

Susceptibility: the relative vulnerability of a specific microorganism to the toxic effects of a tested concentration of an antibiotic.

Susceptible organism: a microorganism subject to the toxic effects of a given concentration of an antibiotic.

Synergism: the ability of one antibiotic to enhance the effect of another.

Ticarcillin: an injectable penicillin particularly effective against bacterial sepsis and infections caused by gram-negative bacteria, notably *Pseudomonas.*

Tobramycin: an aminoglycoside antibiotic particularly effective against *Pseudomonas, Proteus,* and *Klebsiella* infections, but which has potential toxicity for both the ear and kidney.

Tolerance: the ability of a bacterium to withstand otherwise toxic levels of an antibiotic, usually without undergoing growth during exposure.

Transduction: the process whereby genetic material is carried from one bacterium to another by a virus or viruslike agent.

Transformation: genetic change resulting from genetic material being directly incorporated into a bacterial cell's chromosome.

Trimethoprim: a folic acid-inhibiting antibiotic commonly combined with sulfamethoxazole, another folic acid antagonist, as a means of generating synergism.

Turbidity: a measurement of the number of bacteria in a given suspension based on their ability to block the transmission of light.

Vaccine: a suspension, intended either for injection or oral ingestion, of infectious agents or their parts for the purpose of generating resistance to an infectious disease.

Virulence: the relative power or degree of pathogenicity of an organism to produce disease.

Virus: a minute, sub-light-microscopic organism requiring the presence of living cells in which to reproduce and metabolize that can cause infectious diseases in cells or organisms which they parasitize.

Index